Prostate Cancer
Unmasked

Ray M. Schilling, MD

Prostate Cancer Unmasked
Ray M. Schilling, MD

Copyright © 2017 by Ray M. Schilling, MD
All Rights Reserved

Book and Cover Design by Karoline Butler

ISBN-10: 1542880661
ISBN-13: 978-1542880664
Library of Congress Control Number: 2017902174
CreateSpace Independent Publishing Platform
North Charleston, South Carolina

Foreword

With regard to prostate cancer the medical profession has failed its patients.

You hear trumpeted now the importance of "evidence based medicine" and about clinical approaches that are rigorously tested in comparative randomly controlled trials. But the prostate cancer medical community has still not produced a trial comparing the two most often performed prostate cancer treatments, radiation and radical prostatectomy! There would have been a golden opportunity to compare the two radical prostatectomies, namely the Robotic Radical Prostatectomy as being superior to the conventional open or laparoscopic Radical Prostatectomy. But the urologic community preferred not to know the definitive answer to the validation question, which of the two is better. Unfortunately, this lack of comparative data extends through much of the prostate cancer landscape.

Even, however, when the rare study producing level 1 evidence does exist, the results are often ignored, when the preferred clinical approach is not proven to be the superior approach. For instance, Donnelly published the results of a randomized controlled trial in the journal "Cancer", (the journal of the American Cancer Society). He compared whole gland cryoablation with external beam radiation. It showed that cryoablation had a 20% better chance of resulting in negative post treatment biopsies (translating into better cures). While this VERY important information is now known, it has not changed anything. In fact, the use of external beam radiation compared to cryoablation actually increased, due to the economic forces pushing patients toward the money making radiation therapy.

I have experienced this disturbing scenario as a researcher myself. In 2009, we published an article in the Journal of Clinical Oncology (the most prestigious cancer journal in the world) that compared TRUS biopsy (transrectal ultrasound guided biopsy) with a 3D transperineal mapping biopsy. Our results showed beyond a shadow of a doubt that the 3D Mapping biopsy was safer and produced results that could change the management in 70% of prostate cancer patients in a positive fashion. Other investigators have since reproduced the study with the same results. Unfortunately, the 3D-Mapping biopsy, although superior, is only applied in a handful of institutions. At this point the urology community is rejecting it for reasons that relate to physician convenience and reimbursement.

It is the above situation that makes the book "Prostate Cancer Unmasked" of such great value. Dr. Schilling can be a trusted guide to wade through all of the confusing contradictory information out there, so that the prostate cancer patient can make a reasonably informed decision.

"Prostate Cancer Unmasked" is a unique book in a number of ways.

Firstly, the author has a life and career experience, unlike any other authors of a prostate cancer book. Dr. Ray Schilling has had experience as a cancer researcher and as a practicing physician with a long experience seeing prostate cancer patients diagnosed and treated. He has also experienced BEING a prostate cancer patient. He himself had to wade through all the conflicting information regarding various treatments, their possibility of success and the potential impacts they could have on him and his wife's life.

Christina Schilling's input, as a wife of a prostate cancer patient, brings an important perspective to the book. As I have learned treating prostate cancer patients for the last 25 years, this is a disease that impacts a COUPLE, and the decisions regarding the treatment choice are best made as a team. Christina's input in the book provides help for the spouse that has to deal with these decisions as well.

As a result the information you are getting in this book is unlike any other. Many of the books about prostate cancer are written by physicians who treat prostate cancer. This often results in the author pushing his/her own agenda. (Yes, I have my book out there as well!!!) The Schillings have no other agenda than to help other patients and couples navigate the difficult prostate cancer landscape and emerge with a solution that works for them.

"Prostate Cancer Unmasked" is also unique due to the fact that it takes a courageous stand against much of the accepted "wisdom" of prostate cancer establishment. Policy decisions made by politicians and "thought leaders", based on costs and statistics, often lose sight of the plight of the individual patient. As I often have told my patients, "if you are the one person out of a hundred that gets a certain bad result, you don't care that ninety-nine others DIDN'T get it." In this vein Dr. Schilling elucidates why the move away from PSA screening and the move towards a passive management strategy of "active surveillance" may be placing the lives of many patients at risk.

In regard to prostate cancer, the reliance on radical treatments with high morbidity and questionable long-term results and the move toward a passive strategy has led to the abandonment of the basic tenets of cancer therapy:

1. Find it early.
2. Stage it as accurately as possible.
3. Treat it aggressively, appropriate to its stage and tumor aggressiveness.

"Prostate Cancer Unmasked" shows us to be in a paradoxical situation. Early detection of prostate cancer has become difficult, if not impossible, due to new guidelines against routine PSA screening. Why did the U.S. Preventive Services Task Force, a volunteer panel of medical professionals, rule against the wide use of a simple and effective screening tool? Firstly, because men with suspicious or rising test results then underwent an unpleasant and now considered dangerous diagnostic procedure (TRUS biopsy), that has been proven to miss up to 30% of cancers. Those with negative biopsies often have repeat biopsies, with the expenses (anxiety), and complications mounting up. Secondly, because prostate cancer treatments can be highly morbid, it was felt that we were finding too many less aggressive cancers—and the cure was worse than the disease.

A dilemma between over treatment or no treatment occurs when patients diagnosed with low-to-moderate risk cancer are counseled to defer treatment in favor of active surveillance, a strategy for which many patients don't have the psychological tolerance. They worry that a time bomb is ticking in their bodies! Yet they are given this well-intended advice, so they can hold off on the risks of urinary and sexual side effects of whole-gland treatment. So, we don't go looking for cancer because we might find it, overtreat it, and damage men's quality of life? This does not sound logical! Can you think of any other cancer for which early detection is discouraged? It is extremely rare to suggest that other cancers (breast, liver, lung, kidney, liver, etc.) can be safely watched and monitored!

Dr. Schilling has pointed out in this book:

First, there is an alternative to TRUS biopsy that does not involve puncturing the rectal wall and gives extraordinarily accurate tissue diagnosis with no pain and zero risk of septic infection. It is the 3D Mapping Transperineal biopsy (3D-PMB), which is more disease-specific, especially for moderate disease, than MRI-guided targeted biopsies. It improves prostate cancer management decisions by up to 70%. It allows the aggression of the treatment to be matched to that of the disease, and it provides specific localization of the cancer to accurately target the cancer. In short, it meets the first and second tenets of cancer therapy.

Second, an effective FDA-approved minimally invasive procedure is available that satisfies the third tenet of cancer therapy to the major benefit of the prostate cancer patient. That is focal therapy of prostate cancer (i.e. a male lumpectomy) using cryoablation. As Dr. Schilling points out, this has the potential to give better long-term cancer results, while markedly lowering the chance of complications.

I first presented this idea in a 2002 paper demonstrating that we could effectively locate and target a prostate tumor without having to destroy, remove or irradiate the whole gland. By isolating and treating just the tumor and a surrounding safety margin we generate competitive (actually better) efficacy in controlling cancer while preserving healthy tissue to markedly lower morbidity (side effects).

That paper started the ball rolling, and now focal prostate cancer therapy is being carried out in some manner in all the major U.S. cancer centers, including MD Anderson, Johns Hopkins, Sloan Kettering, Duke, and NYU, to name a few. Textbooks have been written on the subject, and at least three major annual medical meetings on this topic are convened each year. The results consistently confirm lower morbidity (side effects) with good cancer control. Dr. Schilling's book is the first to show how this treatment concept can be integrated into a logical approach to prostate cancer treatment.

Finally with an effective low morbidity treatment the pendulum should swing back to early appropriate prostate cancer treatment.

This is an important book, which can save the lives and the life styles of many patients. The education it provides should make each patient comfortable that they have been exposed to the key information they need, before making what is one of the most important decisions in their lives.

Gary Onik, MD
Adjunct Professor of Mechanical Engineering
Carnegie Mellon University
Center for High Risk and Recurrent Prostate Cancer
Ft. Lauderdale, FL
April 2017

Acknowledgments

First, I like to thank my wife, Christina Schilling for contributing to this book. To my friend Gary Onik MD, for his professional input. Last, thanks to Karoline Butler for the book and cover design and help with the publication process.

Dedication

I dedicate this book to all those who have been diagnosed with prostate cancer and to those who are close to them. I hope that it will clarify a lot of the issues surrounding diagnosis and treatment of this illness.

Contents

My Background

Training in Medicine

I had completed my medical training in a traditional medical school in Germany (Tübingen University). After a rotating internship in Tübingen University's teaching hospitals I relocated to Canada and spent a bit more than 3 years doing cancer research at the Ontario Cancer Institute at the Princess Margaret Hospital, Toronto, Ontario. It has since been renamed "The Princess Margaret Cancer Centre".

Despite my fascination with the scientific aspect of medicine, I missed the human aspect and the practical application of medicine. As a result I returned back to medical school at McMaster University in Hamilton, Ontario where I got introduced to the problem-oriented approach to medicine and passed the Canadian State examination (the LMCC exam).

Medical practice as a general practitioner

I started to practice medicine in my family practice in a small town of Southern British Columbia. As I looked after patients over the years I noticed that very often the health problems of the aging population was a study of human suffering. In the 1980's prevention had not become the buzzword that was in everybody's mouth. I knew about vitamin supplements and recommended vitamin E for heart health, which resulted in snarky remarks from some of my more conservative older colleagues. I ignored these remarks, as I had come to the conclusion that prevention of any disease was crucial, before it could wreak havoc with the health of a patient. Over the sixteen years of my family practice in Langley, B.C. I believed in prevention. I encouraged my patients to do everything that was known at the time to prevent obesity, high blood pressure and manage stress through relaxation techniques. It was gratifying to see success!

But cancer was different. It suddenly struck in my patient population, and often it came without a warning. Before colonoscopies were done on a large scale, a patient would suddenly come down with a case of abdominal pain and vomiting. When I referred this patient to a general surgeon, I had to assist with the laparotomy. Often it turned out that a patient had developed bowel obstruction due to colon cancer. This had to be surgically removed, and a temporary colostomy was placed. This is an opening through the skin where the one end of the colon is sown to, which allows stool to be collected in a pouch. A few months later an end-to-end-anastomosis was done, which means the two ends of the colon are sown back together.

Another time a patient that presented first with lower back pain was unmasked as prostate cancer with blood tests and a CT scan of the spine clearly depicting the metastases. Unfortunately we came too late with the diagnosis. This has all changed with mass screening in the 1990's where PSA tests can help to diagnose prostate cancer much earlier.

Medical Advisor for WorkSafeBC

From 1994 until my retirement in 2010 was the second phase of my career where I dealt with occupational medicine (WorkSafeBC of British Columbia). It was often obvious how problematic lifestyles paved the way to arthritic changes and back problems. In these cases prevention was too late, and the only choice was conventional curative medicine. I was still involved in treating patients in a walk- in clinic setting. However, there was a time constraint in examining and talking to patients. Yet it was very clear that patients had questions that could not be dealt with in a 5 to 10 minute visit.

My next projects became two medical websites that would be accessible to everybody and give medical inform-ation in everyday language. This is how www.nethealthbook. com and also a medical blog, www.askdrray.com were started. The first one (www.nethealthbook.com) is a medical data base, where you can find answers to medical topics. The second website (www.askdrray.com) is a collection of blogs on anti-aging topics.

Interest in anti-aging medicine

I learnt more about medical research at conferences for continuing medical education, but there were also new pathways in medicine. A small group of physicians had founded the A4M, the American Academy of Anti Aging Medicine. The number of the A4M members increased dramatically over the years to 26,000 physicians in 2013. I joined them as a member in 2008. I became curious about the conferences that were organized by A4M, and I have since attended their annual A4M conferences.

How I faced prostate cancer

Following the 2015 A4M conference in Las Vegas I decided to order the Oncoblot test as a screening tool for cancer. My mother had died of colon cancer at the age 59. My own physician told me he was observing my borderline high PSA value of 3.0 ng/ml closely. Of course I wondered whether the Oncoblot test would show any markers indicative of prostate or bowel cancer.

To my surprise the Oncoblot test came back "positive for prostate cancer". But there was no sign of colon cancer.

This was a game changer for me. I had to do a lot of research and check out which of the 9 different prostate cancer-treating methods that I could find was right for me. In this book I have done the same review for you, so you can compare the various methods for yourself.

I came to the conclusion that the mapping biopsy followed by cryoablation therapy would be best for me. The mapping biopsy was done July 11, 2016 and this was followed by the cryoablation therapy on Aug. 17, 2016. I am glad that everything went well and that the first follow-up PSA 3 months after the surgery was low (0.9 ng/ml). The Oncoblot test was also repeated 3 months after the surgery and was negative for prostate cancer. Based on this I have a good chance of staying prostate cancer free for at least the next 10 years.

Not all of my questions about prostate cancer were answered. Since 2001 I followed a very healthy diet and I had cut out sugar and starchy foods. I exercise regularly in a gym. I apply all the things I hear at A4M conferences that I find useful. And yet I came down with prostate cancer! But this is how life is. We need to accept and deal with it and continue living. Unfortunately we cannot control everything by a good lifestyle.

I am sure that I am not the only man on this planet who wonders why he was "chosen" to get this disease.

While I was staying in a hotel room in Ft. Lauderdale waiting for my prostate surgery, I got the idea that I should write a book for those who like me have to face that they have prostate cancer. You may have had a prostate biopsy that was positive or you had a PSA test that came back high. This will automatically raise the question of what you should do next?

I hope that with the information in this book you will find what fits you best.

Don't despair; don't get intimidated by health professionals, just soldier on. But whatever you do, do not accept that "active surveillance" should be an option. As I discussed in the book, when men accept active surveillance their mortality rate is 50% higher than if they choose active treatment at the time of diagnosis. The facts, which I have gathered in this book, are a tool for you to inform yourself and to help you fight for your rights. This may require a change in health professionals. The road is not always smooth, but it worked for me. It is my hope that it works for you as well!

Introduction

There have been many books written about prostate cancer. You may ask why I wrote another book about this topic. You will see below that I am suggesting a different approach to treating prostate cancer. Any prostate cancer should be taken seriously, and there is no room for "active surveillance".

Prostate cancer is a topic that has been close to my heart, as I have seen many patients in my general practice die of this disease. I hoped then that one time in the future there would be a better way to treat this cancer.

In the beginning of my practice there was no prostate-specific antigen (PSA) screening test available, only rectal examinations. As patients with prostate cancer were often older men, the urologist decided to just do a TURP (transurethral resection of the prostate) to help patients with urination problems to urinate again. But the prostate cancer was not eradicated. Invariably the prostate cancer patients came back complaining about dribbling. The TURP procedure is now thought of as archaic. Urologists always thought about my patients differently from what I believed in. They thought that patients with prostate cancer were older and they may be more in danger of dying of a heart attack or a stroke rather than from their prostate cancer. Based on this thought they just did the minimum procedure that had to be done rather than to attempt to cure the prostate cancer.

As you can tell from the title "Prostate Cancer Unmasked", I think about this disease differently. I wanted my patients to get a cure from their prostate cancer. Fortunately the FDA approved the PSA test in 1986 as a "monitor for treatment response and disease recurrence". Later in 1994 the FDA approved the PSA test as a screening tool for prostate cancer. Finally a sensitive and fairly specific test for prostate cancer has become available (the Oncoblot test)! But the question remained: what was the best treatment tool?

I am reviewing 9 different treatment approaches in this book. They are all currently in use by different physicians. But they do not necessarily serve the patient best. In my opinion effective treatment is necessary in order to achieve a cure. Brachytherapy does not quite do it. It improves the cancer for a period of time, and after a few years it returns with a vengeance. The radical prostatectomy and the robotic prostatectomy have helped a significant amount of patients. But long-term studies show that there can be a recurrence rate of as much as 25 to 30%. In addition there are significant side effects like a killed sex life and involuntary dribbling of urine, if the bladder outlet was injured during the surgery. Quite often urologists recommend "active surveillance". This mysterious approach to prostate cancer means that a 71 to 75 year old prostate cancer sufferer is kept in suspense by the urologist. An initial rectal biopsy is done with a histology assessment where a Gleason score is analyzed. If this score is 6 or less, the cancer is presumed to be less aggressive and active surveillance is done. If the Gleason score is 7 or higher it means the tumor is more aggressive and the urologist will decide to treat it. If the score is in the lower range, another biopsy is done 1 year later and this could go on until the patient dies of a heart attack or a stroke. This was the original reasoning, namely that the urologist did not want to do an invasive prostate surgery in someone who might die from another disease.

I have never heard that active surveillance is done in any of the other cancers. It used to be called "watchful waiting". Maybe too many people nicknamed this "watchful neglect", after which it was renamed "active surveillance". Fact is that I have seen patients where active surveillance backfired, and the prostate cancer had taken off like any other cancer does.

I think that prostate cancer should be treated early before metastases develop and the cancer gets out of control. There are other methods that actually can get rid of the prostate cancer, for instance cryoablation therapy following a mapping biopsy. In this latter method 60 biopsies are placed like a grid through the entire prostate gland to identify the exact location where prostate cancer has developed. This is done through the perineum (between the scrotum and the anal opening). Prostate cancer can often be multifocal: there may be two or three areas where prostate cancer is located. One month after the mapping procedure probes are introduced in the same way, through the perineum and the identified cancer lesions are treated with cryotherapy twice. I am explaining this in chapter 15 in more detail.

According to Dr. Onik, an interventional radiologist in Ft. Lauderdale, active surveillance is something that should be abandoned. Instead the following treatment approach should be adopted.

1. A rising PSA or single PSA above 30 should trigger a referral for a mapping biopsy through the perineal approach under a general anesthetic. The treating physician can sterilize the area and perform biopsies in

a sterile fashion, which prevents infection. This is a huge advantage above the standard transrectal approach, which can lead to infections like prostatitis and blood poisoning.

2. Based on the result of the mapping biopsy targeted ablation cryotherapy is performed one month later eradicating all the cancer foci determined through the mapping biopsy.

3. Follow-up PSA levels are obtained every three months for 2 years. If the PSA is less than 3.0, the patient is considered cured. If there is a rising PSA level point 1 and 2 above are repeated until a cure is achieved.

This treatment approach is the same for early prostate cancer patients or for advanced cases. Dr. Gary Onik published a 10-year follow-up study that had a 100% survival rate and a 94% cure rate in 70 men with prostate cancer.

The reason for such good results is that attention is paid to detail, to the exact location of the cancer and that all cancer is completely eradicated. In my opinion this is the new blueprint of a common sense approach to prostate cancer. Read more details about this in chapter 15. But I am also reviewing the gold standard of the radical prostatectomy in its various forms (suprapubic conventional surgery, laparoscopic and robotic surgery). In addition I reviewed brachytherapy, external beam radiotherapy, laser ablation therapy and high-intensity focused ultrasound treatment. I noticed that the long-term cure rates over 10 years differ considerably from one treatment modality to the next. All of this is reviewed in detail in this book, so you can make up your own mind what is best for you.

About This Book

Here I am briefly summarizing what each chapter of this book is about.

Chapter 1. When Prostate Cancer Did Not Kill

Before the PSA test was invented, the only test for prostate cancer was the digital rectal exam. Unfortunately prostate cancer was often diagnosed at a late stage. But life expectancy in the 1960's was only about 65, and men would often die from heart attacks or strokes before prostate cancer killed them.

Chapter 2. The PSA Test

I am reviewing the history of the PSA test and how physicians have been using the test. Health regulators try to discourage using this test, as they say too many cases of prostate cancer are diagnosed with it. Don't get sidetracked by this point of view. I explain why.

Chapter 3. A Brief Anatomy Lesson & Prostate Biopsy

I felt that a brief reminder of the location of the prostate gland and connection to other organs in the region would be useful. This explains why complications with the gold standard of the radical prostatectomy can lead to urinary incontinence, bowel incontinence and erectile dysfunction. Next a prostate biopsy has to be done, if the PSA is high. The problems with a rectal biopsy and the advantages of a mapping biopsy are reviewed.

Chapter 4. Staging of Prostate Cancer & Genetic Changes

It is important for the treating physician or urologist to assess how far spread the prostate cancer is. This requires a comprehensive accumulation of data like the tumor location and possible lymph node metastases, seen on MRI scan and ultrasound imaging. The height of the PSA is needed. Tests are also establishing whether there are other metastases in distant organs. This information determines what the outlook is for this patient (prognosis). All of this information determines what treatment modalities need to be employed. In the second half of this chapter I give a brief review about what is known regarding the genetics of prostate cancer.

Chapter 5. A Silent Killer

A patient drops into my office with a low back pain and is sent for blood tests and X-rays. He has metastatic disease. All tests turn out horrible; he dies not long after from end stage prostate cancer.

Chapter 6. Help Comes Too Late

Fred is a patient who is found to have a hard mass on rectal examination. His PSA is 15. The urologist biopsies and confirms prostate cancer. He is being treated with radiotherapy, which gives him 4 good years. But then trouble starts.

Chapter 7. Stop the Hormones – But Does it Stop Cancer?

When radiotherapy or a prostatectomy has been done and the prostate cancer returns, it seems like a knee-jerk reaction to do hormone ablation therapy. I am discussing here what testosterone really does. I am explaining that the basic assumption that testosterone would make prostate cancer worse or that it would be the cause for it has been wrong all along.

Chapter 8. Active Surveillance for "A Little Bit of Cancer"

This is a very popular concept in North America. But it has been abandoned in Sweden and Denmark, because the Cancer Agencies there found that too many people died needlessly while medical personnel did "active surveillance". The opposite is true: you need to intervene and treat prostate cancer early. For instance, if you do a mapping biopsy and ablation cryotherapy shortly after, you likely will kill all prostate cancer cells and cure the cancer early.

Chapter 9. Detected in Time

A 75-year-old relative of mine was detected to have prostate cancer because of a high PSA and a positive prostate biopsy. The urologist suggested radiotherapy, but I explained to my relative that the long-term survival rates are poor. I suggested to him to have a nerve sparing radical prostatectomy done instead (the gold standard). He did well with this procedure and is now 89 years old.

Chapter 10. Radical Prostatectomy a Success?

The original prostatectomy was the open procedure, which was subsequently modified into a laparoscopic prostatectomy, a closed procedure where laparoscopic instruments are used instead. In order to minimize erectile dysfunction the highly selective prostatectomy was invented, which pays particular attention to preserving the neurovascular bundle on each side of the prostate. Sometimes the prostate cancer reaches close to the neurovascular bundles. In these cases it is likely that the surgeon has to remove one or both of them, and this causes severe erectile dysfunction. Urinary incontinence is the other big complication, when the surgeon gets too close to the bladder neck. Nevertheless this surgery is still being called the "gold standard". But the laparoscopic prostatectomy, according to a Johns Hopkins study only has a 10- year survival rate of 77%. Compare this to Dr. Onik's ablation cryotherapy with a 10-year survival rate of 100%; 94% of the patients were completely free from any recurring prostate cancer and 6% had recurring disease.

Chapter 11. The Robotic Revolution

This form of radical prostatectomy is using robotic equipment to do the same what an open prostatectomy or a laparoscopic prostatectomy would achieve. The only difference is that it may leave less tissue damage behind, as the robotic equipment uses miniaturized tools that are controlled from a computerized remote console. Healing rates are about the same, but complications like urinary incontinence, bowel incontinence and erectile dysfunction may be less common.

Chapter 12. Radiation, Brachytherapy & Proton Therapy

Radiation and brachytherapy may help in the short term for up to 4 or 5 years. But the 10-year survival data revealed a sad picture as only 57% of patients survived that long after a combination of brachytherapy and radiotherapy when their prostate cancer was treated by the Georgia Center for Prostate Cancer Research. Another form of radiotherapy, the more gentle, but very expensive proton therapy had a 10-year survival rate of 73%. Low risk patients with an initial PSA of less than 4 had a 10-year survival rate of 90%.

Chapter 13. Intervention with Laser - The Light of Hope?

Laser treatment sounds like new technology, which it is. There are high-energy lasers that can leave more scarring, and there are low-dose lasers. When low-dose lasers are combined with radio sensitizers, they can kill esophagus cancer and lung cancer. But prostate cancer treatment has not yet been perfected. I could not find any 10-year survival rates for low-dose or high-dose laser therapy. Laser treatment for prostate cancer is considered to be highly experimental at this stage.

Chapter 14. A Woman's View of Prostate Cancer

My wife, Christina described how she felt when I was diagnosed with prostate cancer. She also tells you about the agony to decide, which procedure to use to get rid of it. We settled on Dr. Onik's ablation cryotherapy discussed in the next chapter. She managed to verbalize all of the thought processes we went through as a couple.

Chapter 15. Ablation Cryotherapy after Mapping Biopsy

Before ablation cryotherapy can be done, the patient needs a mapping biopsy, where the whole prostate gland is methodically biopsied every 5 mm, until the entire prostate has been biopsied. This takes 60 to 90 needles depending on the size of the prostate and is called a mapping biopsy. The ablation cryotherapy is done under rectal ultrasound guidance. It is performed in the exact same areas where the previous mapping biopsy was done. The approach is through the perineum, which eliminates the risk of infection, as the perineum can be kept sterile. In a clinical trial of 70 prostate cancer patients there was a 100% survival of the prostate cancer patients treated with cryotherapy. 94% were completely free from any recurring prostate cancer 10 years after treatment, 6% had recurring disease. The percentage of complications like urinary incontinence, rectal incontinence or erectile dysfunction were a fraction, when compared to the other surgical or radiological treatment methods.

Chapter 16. Chemotherapy of Prostate Cancer

Both radiotherapy and chemotherapy lead to resistant prostate cancer cells. The reason is that prostate cancer stem cells are resistant to both chemotherapy and radiotherapy. This is why cure rates are so disappointing with all of these treatment methods.

Chapter 17. Prostate Cancer Stem Cells

Until recently nobody knew that prostate cancer stem cells existed. However, there are several mouse models with which human prostate cancer stem cells can be injected and human prostate cancer grows in the mice that were injected, if stem cells were present. This literature is reviewed in this chapter. It is also mentioned that only prostatectomy, ablation cryotherapy and IRE surgery (which is explained) will remove prostate cancer stem cells. This is why the cure rates with ablation cryotherapy are much higher. The concept of cancer immunotherapy is also explained.

Chapter 18. Prevention of Prostate Cancer

There are several factors that can help prevent prostate cancer. Vitamin D3 intake will reduce the prostate cancer rate, even in patients of African background who ordinarily have twice the risk of getting prostate cancer. Get rid of the beer belly, because it manufactures estrogen causing prostate cancer. A healthy balanced nutrition like a Mediterranean diet is also important for prevention.

Chapter 19. Differential Diagnosis: Prostatitis & Benign Prostatic Hyperplasia (BPH)

There are other conditions of the prostate gland that are important to know about. Two of these common conditions are prostatitis and BPH. Here I am describing them in detail. They do not cause prostate cancer, but it is important to know about them as all three conditions, prostate cancer, prostatitis and BPH affect the same prostate gland.

Chapter 20. Prostate Cancer Support Groups

I am providing a link to a website where you find prostate cancer support groups. But I am also cautioning you not to get dependent on their advice. You want to use them to broaden your knowledge about prostate cancer. But you don't want to use them to be railroaded into what everybody else is doing. It is not true that a prostatectomy is the gold standard to treat prostate cancer anymore; ablation cryotherapy is the gold standard in the meantime, but many support groups have not heard about that. Also in this chapter is a brief summary of what to do in the case of advanced prostate cancer disease.

Chapter 21. Conclusion: What Does It Mean to Unmask Prostate Cancer?

After the overview of all the treatment modalities for prostate cancer I urge the reader to judge each method by its 10-year survival rates. You need a yardstick by which you can measure the success or failure rate of any treatment method. Dr. Onik's ablation cryotherapy is the only one of the reviewed treatment methods that has a survival rate of 100% at the 10-year follow-up point. 94% of the treated patients were completely free from any recurring prostate cancer. Only 6% had recurrent cancer. In those patients the mapping biopsy could be repeated and another ablation cryotherapy treatment could be done. Every effort was taken that all website links quoted in this book were functioning properly at the time of publishing. However, due to updates or changes they may result in broken links.

Ray M. Schilling, MD
Kelowna, BC, Canada
April 2017

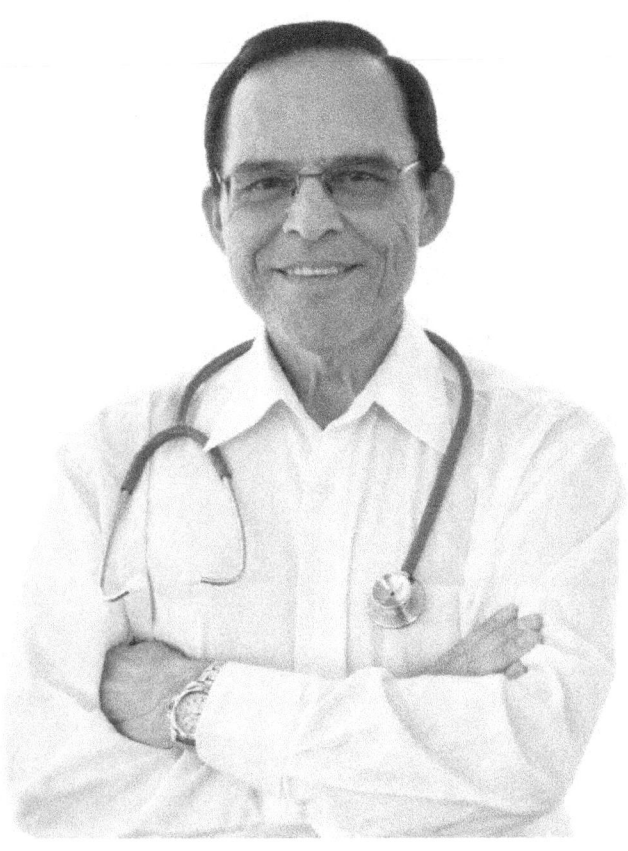

Ray M. Schilling, MD - 2017

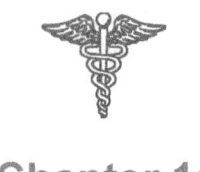

Chapter 1

When Prostate Cancer Did Not Kill

It is not long ago that life expectancy for men was only 65 to 68 years. This was the case in the 1960's, and it was mainly heart attacks and strokes that were the major killers.

Prostate cancer is the most common cancer in males apart from skin cancer. In the US there were 180,890 new prostate cancer cases diagnosed in 2016. In the same year about 26,120 died from prostate cancer. About 1 man in 7 will be diagnosed with prostate cancer in his lifetime. 60% of prostate cancer patients are 65 years or older when the diagnosis is made. Prostate cancer is rare to occur before the age of 40. Prostate cancer can be a serious disease, but most men do not die from it. More than 2.9 million men who have been diagnosed with prostate cancer are still alive today. About 1 man in 39 will die of prostate cancer. It is the second leading cause of death in men behind lung cancer.

http://www.cancer.org/cancer/prostatecancer/detailedguide/prostate-cancer-key-statistics

Prostate cancer is a cancer that grows slowly and stays within a tough capsule, so it is often still an early stage when an elevated PSA level is found. If the cancer is left alone, the patient may die only 10 or 15 years later. This is why urologists came up with the "active surveillance" scheme. But today men can turn 80 or 85, and they don't want to be bothered about prostate cancer giving them bone pains and making them die prematurely. With proper life styling (eating a Mediterranean type diet, exercising regularly, cutting out sugar and not smoking) you could turn 90 to 95 or older. Why should you not have your prostate cancer removed at the age of 75, if your PSA level is high at that time and the biopsy confirms prostate cancer? In the past an outdated treatment method was a TURP, if the patient could not pass urine. But the cancer was left in place. Today the proper procedure is to do a perineal mapping biopsy and follow this up with ablation cryotherapy, once the exact pathology is known. This way all of the cancer cells are removed. 10 years later 100% of patients are still alive and in 94% of cases all of the cancer is still gone; 6 % of cases would have a recurrence, which can be treated again with ablation surgery.

But urologists up to this day insist that they want to do active surveillance in a patient with a low-grade prostate cancer rather than do a prostatectomy. They also still argue that a 75-year-old male with prostate cancer will not live long enough to die from the prostate cancer, but rather will likely die from a heart attack or a stroke. I find this irresponsible. As we will see later the Cancer Control Agencies in Sweden and in Denmark also don't agree with this concept. To the opposite: they suggest immediate treatment with radiation or surgery in any prostate cancer case as their huge collection of data shows a 50% better long- term survival rate when active surveillance is bypassed and definite cancer treatment is used instead.

Conclusion

There was a time up to 1960 to 1970 when the male life expectancy was so short that prostate cancer appeared to not shorten a man's life. But with the life expectancy now being in the mid 80's things have changed. It is no longer true that we can leave prostate cancer alone as "he will die of a heart attack or of stroke first". The earlier he notices that his PSA is increased, the earlier a mapping biopsy can be done, the faster he will recover from ablation cryotherapy or any other surgical method.

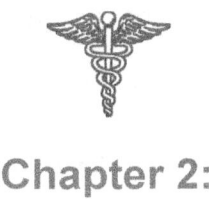

Chapter 2

The PSA Test

The FDA approved PSA testing as a tool for early prostate cancer screening in 1994. Prior to that the only way to diagnose prostate cancer was a digital rectal examination. When prostate cancer was diagnosed this way, in 50% of cases men had already metastatic disease. Now with the PSA blood test only 5% of men with prostate cancer have metastatic disease at the time of diagnosis. The test is so sensitive that the idea of "watchful waiting" or "active surveillance" was coined to manage the many non-invasive prostate cancers and filter out the cancers that are more aggressive. As I mentioned before the problem with this concept is that a sizable portion of men will miss the point where the cancer invades the neighboring structures. By the time the urologist notices that the cancer is getting more aggressive, metastases have already occurred. This increases the relapse rate when a radical prostatectomy or radiotherapy treatment is done. At that time you would want to go back in time, but you can't. It is too late and the outlook is bleak.

Here are a few facts about PSA:

- With every year a healthy adult man increases the PSA level by 0.04 ng/ml

- After a radical prostatectomy the PSA should go down to 0.2 ng/ml or less
- If following a prostatectomy the PSA goes above 0.4 ng/ml suspect cancer recurrence
- For screening purposes, if a man has a PSA level of 2.5 ng/ml, test yearly as some men may develop a further rise, which then requires a prostate biopsy to look for prostate cancer
- With a PSA level of 4.0 ng/ml the patient should be referred to a urologist for a prostate biopsy
- A man with a family history of prostate cancer should be referred to a urologist if his PSA level has risen to values from 2.5 ng/ml to 4.0ng/ml

The PSA story is further complicated by the fact that prostatitis can raise the PSA by a factor of 5- to 7-fold. Urinary retention will do the same. Benign hypertrophy of the prostate (BPH) can increase the PSA up to 10 ng/ml. Sitting on a bike and exercising can increase the PSA 3-fold. A cystoscopy can elevate the PSA 4- fold. A prostate biopsy and a TURP (transurethral resection of the prostate) can elevate the PSA 50-fold. The half-life of the PSA is three days. So it could take between 10 and 40 days after these procedures for PSA levels to return back to normal. The treating physician must take all of these factors into account before concluding that an elevated PSA may be due to prostate cancer. The definite test to diagnose prostate cancer is a prostate biopsy, but you do not want to do this to a patient, if he has been riding an exercise bike regularly. It makes sense to advise him to stop riding the bike and wait 40 days before having a PSA blood test repeated.

When to screen with the PSA test

The Prostate Cancer Advisory Committee of the American Cancer Society (ACS) said this: "Prostate cancer screening should not occur without an informed discussion about risks and benefits."

The ACS gave the following age suggestions for PSA testing:
- Start at age 50 for men with an average risk
- Start at age 45 for men with a higher risk. This includes African American men and men who have a father or brother that was diagnosed with prostate cancer before the age of 65
- Start at age 40 years for men with an appreciably higher risk; this includes those with multiple family members who had prostate cancer before the age of 65. PSA monitoring has made a big difference in the lives of older men. There are options of long-term survival now, where there was despair in the past.

PSA velocity and free PSA

The urologist may determine the PSA velocity and also order a free PSA level. Both are tests that can make an increased PSA level more prostate cancer specific. Let's assume that the PSA range in a patient is in the 4.0- to 10.0 ng/mL range, and the patient has an enlarged prostate due to prostate hyperplasia. If next year's PSA level shows a rise of more than 0.75 ng/mL, this rise would be due to prostate cancer. This PSA velocity has a detection specificity of 90% and a sensitivity of 79%.

The free PSA measures the prostate specific portion of the PSA. Free PSA is expressed as free-to-total PSA as percentage. If this is found to be under 25% this is very likely due to prostate cancer. This is particularly good for PSA levels between 4 and 10 ng/mL, when free PSA can predict 90% of prostate cancers.

http://www.cancernetwork.com/articles/percent-free-psa-test-may-prevent-unnecessary-biopsies

It also allows eliminating 20% of unnecessary biopsies, particularly in older men.

PSA screening for prostate cancer NOT obsolete

Around 2005 there was a strong campaign that too many PSA tests would be run and too many positive test results would be "clogging up" the medical system.

Insurance systems even went so far as to no longer cover this test, so people had to pay for it privately (big deal, it is only in the $20 range).

Like with any test there are false positive results, and the PSA blood test has received some criticism as a result of this. Negative comments likening it to "Shooting flies with a bazooka" have been voiced, and yet, mortality statistics on prostate cancer tell a different story.

20 years ago prostate cancer mortality was 1 in 3 patients. Today the mortality is only 1 in 100 patients.

In the last few years the prostate cancer mortality rate in North America is down by 25%, and part of it is due to the PSA test. If PSA testing would be stopped, prostate cancer mortality would be going back to the bad old times, were men where diagnosed only, once the prostate cancer was advanced, had formed metastases, and hopes for a cure were remote. There are promising new tests under development (the Oncoblot test is already available, but expensive), which at one point in time may replace the PSA test. For now the PSA test is still the best screening test available. The only other way to find prostate cancer is by doing a biopsy.

The Memorial Sloan Kettering Cancer Center has written a sensible recommendation where the younger patients are treated more aggressively than the older ones.

https://www.mskcc.org/cancer-care/types/prostate/
screening/screening-guidelines-prostate

This way the patient is protected from overzealous urological surgeons and the side effects of surgery when surgery may not be indicated.

But the bottom line is that PSA screening is not obsolete. A rising PSA level can only be detected when there was a baseline because of several measurements along the road.

The classical cut-off point for a normal PSA level was below 4.0 ng/mL. But lately many urologists recommend a PSA level below 2.5 ng/mL.

5α-reductase inhibitors (finasteride, dutasteride) lower the PSA within 6 months to 50% of the original level. In these patients the PSA value must be doubled to obtain the true PSA value.

Conclusion

PSA testing has become the cornerstone of good prostate cancer screening. PSA testing is sensitive enough to diagnose prostate cancer early when it is in stage 1 or 2. At this time it can be treated with various treatment modalities. And after treatment is finished, PSA tests serve as a valuable follow-up tool to screen for any possible recurrence of the cancer. If following ablation cryotherapy the PSA rose again, it means that there was a prostate cancer recurrence. In this case the mapping biopsy and the cryotherapy procedure could be repeated. This scenario would be more problematical with other treatment methods due to extensive scarring.

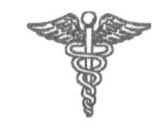

Chapter 3

A Brief Anatomy Lesson & Prostate Biopsy

The prostate gland is situated underneath the bladder within the pelvis of the male. The bases of the swelling bodies (corpora) of the penis are touching the prostate gland from below. The urethra, which is the tube draining urine from the bladder to the outside, goes right through the center of the prostate and the penis. In the back of the prostate is the rectal wall. This is the reason why a bowel movement can cause pain in the prostate following prostate surgery, and this pain can persist for weeks. The prostate is providing 40% of the semen fluid that is ejaculated with sex. The other 60% of fluid comes from the seminal vesicles. These are attached to each side of the prostate from below and have their own ducts that enter the urethra inside the prostate gland. They are important, because with prostate cancer the cancer tissue can metastasize into the seminal vesicles, which makes prostate cancer treatment much more difficult. The testicles are also indirectly connected to the prostate through the vas deferens on each side, which originates in the testicles and ends in the seminal vesicles.

During sex the sperm stored in the seminal vesicles travels through the opening in the prostatic urethra into the prostate, mix with the semen fluid from the prostate gland and get ejaculated into the woman's upper vagina close to the cervix. The cervical canal produces a sperm-friendly mucous, which helps transporting the sperm inside the womb.

You may think that this is a complicated system. I wondered about this too as a medical student. But things are like this and the system works, or there would be no people on planet earth.

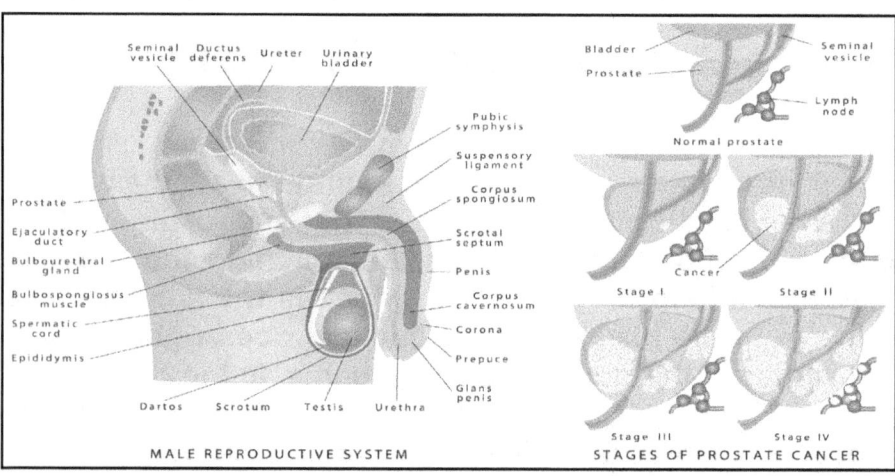

MALE REPRODUCTIVE SYSTEM   STAGES OF PROSTATE CANCER

The inside of the prostate gland has a certain structure that is important to know about, when it comes to the development of prostate cancer. There is a peripheral zone, a central zone and a transition zone. Also there are the neurovascular bundles, one on each side of the prostate gland. 70% of cancers develop in the peripheral zone, the outer area close to the rectum. But prostate cancer often starts not only in one spot, but can start simultaneously in two or three spots. I will describe the facts in chapter 15 how MRI scans may not be infallible and may fail to show all the lesions. The crucial data the doctor needs to know is whether the prostate cancer is close to one or both of the neurovascular bundles. If it is, the techniques will have to be modified by using the NanoKnife (or IRE, all explained in chapter 15), which will not injure the neurovascular bundles. In the center ablation cryotherapy can be used. Caution needs to be exerted around the urethra, which goes through the middle of the prostate.

The anatomy is important when it comes to other surgical treatment methods. With the radical prostatectomy the so-called bladder neck can get injured. This will result in permanent bladder leakage problems (called urinary incontinence) as the double sphincter is not working anymore in keeping urine reliably in the bladder. This can also happen from radiation damage with brachytherapy, radiation therapy or proton radiotherapy. Radiation can also irritate the rectal wall and cause radiation proctitis.

Both surgery and radiation therapy often injure one or both of the neurovascular bundles. This can be very upsetting for a man. It is the difference of not having sex (when injured) or eventually enjoying sex again, once the swelling from the surgery has calmed down. This can also influence urinary control.

Prostate biopsy

When the PSA is elevated, the next step the urologist will suggest is a prostate biopsy. There are two types of prostate biopsies, the conventional transrectal biopsy and the perineal mapping biopsy.

Transrectal prostate biopsy

Typically the physician takes between 6 and 16 random biopsies through the rectum. But this is potentially dangerous, as the rectum contains a lot of bacteria, called Escherichia coli. The gram-negative bacteria can end up in the blood by doing this procedure and cause a dangerous infection, called septicemia.

Septicemia simply means "bugs in your blood". Usually this is treated in the hospital, because it requires an intravenous line and at least two, if not three antibiotics to quickly eliminate the bug from the system. Unfortunately there is a 1 in 200 chance of getting septicemia. To reduce the risk of infection, the patient is usually prepared with pre-operative antibiotics before the procedure.

The other problem with random biopsies is that the specialist does not know where exactly the biopsy came from. And because the biopsies don't represent the entire prostate gland as the mapping biopsy does, there are many areas that can be potentially missed. These negative biopsy results are called "false negatives" as there would be cancer, but it was missed on biopsy. Comparative studies have shown that the success rate of the transrectal biopsy approach is 10% lower than the transperineal approach.

Mapping biopsy of the prostate

There is an alternative, safer way to do a prostate biopsy, the 3-dimensional mapping biopsy of Dr. Onik. In this case the needles are inserted through a brachytherapy grid over the perineum, the skin between the scrotum and the anus. The area can be thoroughly disinfected, which eliminates the risk of infection as the needles are placed. The patient is under a general anesthetic and the specialist inserts between 60 and 90 biopsy needles through the perineum into the prostate gland. This way the entire prostate gland is probed using biopsy needles and no area of cancer is missed. The procedure is watched through a transrectal ultrasound (TRUS) probe. Each of the biopsies is carefully labeled and kept track of, so the results from the pathologist can be entered on a map (hence the name mapping biopsy). This is like a geographical image of the areas where prostate cancer was found. It is not a paper map, but a computer generated ultrasound image of the patient's prostate gland with overlaying histology results. Because of the higher number of biopsy needles used with mapping biopsies the resolution is much better compared to the TRUS guided rectal biopsies. It also tells the treating physician exactly where the cancer is located, if this is going to be treated with ablative cryotherapy.

Diabetic patients who are more prone to infections are preferentially biopsied with this type of perineal prostate mapping biopsy. The advantage is that the perineum can be thoroughly disinfected and there is a very low, if not negligible infection rate following this procedure.

Result of prostate biopsy

Most people think there is only one type of prostate cancer. But when the pathologist analyzes the appearance of the biopsy sample under the microscope about 90% of the samples will be the familiar glandular prostate cancer, medically known as acinar adenocarcinoma. This is what is generally meant when the doctor talks about prostate cancer. It originates from the glandular cell type that produces the fluid that is mixed into the semen. The remaining 10% can be any one of the following 6 types:

- Carcinoid of the prostate. This starts from cells of the neuroendocrine system. It is a very rare type of prostate cancer, can stay dormant for some time, but then takes off rapidly.
- Ductal adenocarcinoma. This type of prostate cancer originates from the ducts of the prostate. This is a type

that grows more rapidly than the acinar adenocarcinoma and spreads more rapidly.

- Sarcoma and sarcomatoid cancers. The leiomyosarcoma is the most common sarcoma. This type of prostate cancer originates from muscle cells that are found throughout the prostate gland. They multiply fast. With sarcomatoid cancers there is a combination of adenocarcinoma cells and sarcoma cells.
- Small cell cancer. This cancer originates from neuroendocrine cells within the prostate. It does not elevate the PSA level, which makes it difficult initially to diagnose. It multiplies more quickly and spreads faster than the regular adenocarcinoma.
- Squamous cell cancer. The flat epithelial cells that cover the prostate gland can turn into this type of prostate cancer. This type of cancer grows faster and spreads more quickly than the regular acinaradenocarcinoma.
- Transitional cell cancer. The cell type that lines the urethra and the inside of the bladder can turn cancerous where it travels through the prostate. It can spread from there into the prostate.

This is all pathologist talk, and it is histological information, which is not that important for the patient to know. But it has some significance for the specialist who treats this patient with any of these other types of prostate cancer. Overall it will not affect too many patients. But those with faster growing, more dangerous subtypes of prostate cancer will not be encouraged to go on a program of "active surveillance", but rather opt for a surgical removal technique (including ablation cryotherapy) or for proton radiotherapy right away.

Conclusion

I reviewed the anatomy of the prostate briefly. It is important to note that any part of the prostate gland can turn cancerous; there are 7 major types of prostate cancer types, where one is common and the other 6 are less common. They all have different inherent stages of aggressiveness. A prostate biopsy will show what type of cancer it is and what Gleason score is present. As will be explained in the next chapter, the higher the numbers of the Gleason score the more aggressive the prostate cancer is. It also matters whether you have random transrectal prostate biopsies or a mapping biopsy. Dr. Onik's mapping biopsy covers the entire prostate gland with a biopsy needle every 5 millimeters. You are less likely to miss any cancer with the mapping biopsy. Dr. Onik has reexamined a number of patients who had radical prostatectomies for prostate cancer. He found with mapping biopsies that their recurrences came from missed cancerous areas in their prostates in their previous random transrectal biopsies.

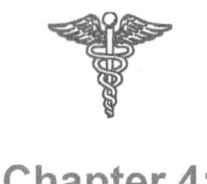

Staging of Prostate Cancer & Genetic Changes

A) Staging of prostate cancer

Overview

Staging of prostate cancer is as important as in other cancers. It allows the physician to assess at which level the cancer is at the time of diagnosis. This process is called staging. It might involve some X rays, perhaps a bone scan and more blood tests, such as an acid phosphatase, which correlates well with the presence of bone metastases. A transrectal ultrasound (TRUS) and a TRUS guided prostate biopsy in at least 6 different areas of the prostate would also be required. The prostate biopsy material can be analyzed by the pathologist according to how well differentiated the cells look under the microscope. A comparison is made between the grading of the normal looking cells and the worst looking prostate cancer cells in the biopsy specimens. These scores are added, and a Gleason score is obtained. The higher the number, the more aggressive the cancer cells are. Mostly scores are in the 6 to 7 (out of 10) Gleason score category. A Gleason 8 (out of 10) score would be a more aggressive prostate cancer.

Finally the doctor may want to employ a CT or MRI scan to delineate any involvement of the cancer outside the prostatic capsule and to determine the size of the prostate cancer.

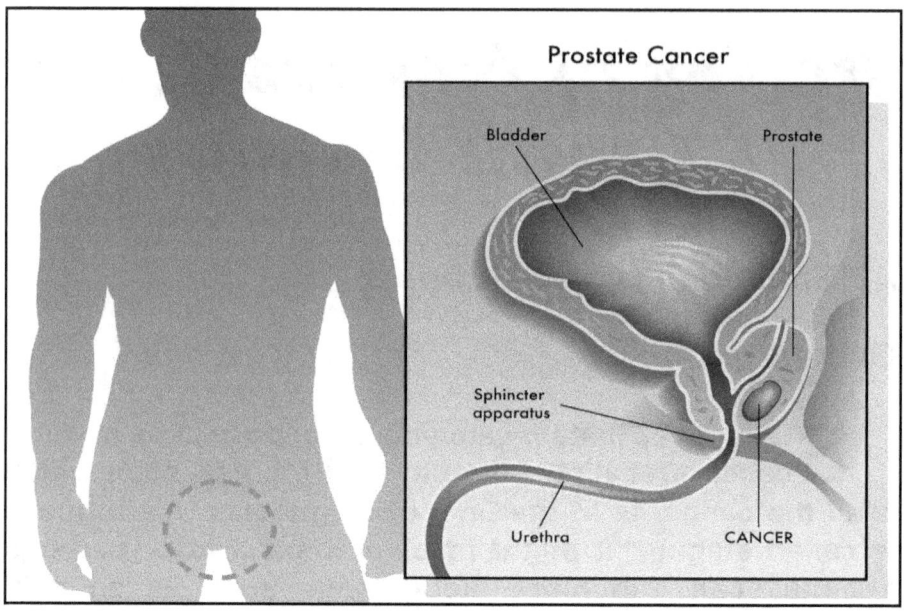

More details

Here are the stages in Roman numerals as suggested by the American Joint Committee on Cancer (AJCC). The AJCC suggests using this for prostate cancer staging.

- *Stage I:* Positive PSA and biopsy confirmed prostate cancer confined to one lobe; clinically not visible by imaging techniques or exam
- *Stage II:* Prostate cancer clinically palpable by rectal exam; visible on TRUS, subclasses confined to one or both lobes
- *Stage III:* Prostate cancer extends through the prostatic capsule with local regional metastases, sometimes with seminal vesicle invasion
- *Stage IV:* The prostate is fixed due to extensive invasion of adjacent structures including the pelvic bone; there may also be distant metastases

The American Joint Committee on Cancer (AJCC) also suggests using the TNM system, which was introduced years ago by the Union for International Cancer Control (UICC).

The TNM system consists of 5 pieces of information that describe how advanced the prostate tumor is (T stands for tumor), whether lymph nodes are involved (N stands for nodes) and whether there are distant metastases (M stands for metastases). It also requires the PSA value and Gleason score from the biopsy.

If you are curious to read through the doctor's report and make sense of the abbreviations, terms and medical lingo, the next passage will demystify some of the terms. It's not an uncomplicated read! I have added it for those who want more in-depth information. If you are not interested in these rather overwhelming intricacies, you may want to skip over the next section!

About the tumor

There are 4 categories as follows.

- *T1:* The doctor can't feel the tumor by rectal examination or find it by transrectal ultrasound study. But a surgical procedure or biopsy has found some cancer cells. There are three subcategories of T1, called *T1a, T1b* and *T1c* depending on how much pathology is found.
- *T2:* The doctor can feel the cancer with a digital rectal exam (DRE) or see a lesion on a transrectal ultrasound. There are three subcategories. *T2a* is used when the prostate cancer is confined to less than one half of one side (left or right) of your prostate gland. *T2b* is used when the tumor is in more than one half of one side of the prostate. *T2c:* The cancer is on both sides of the prostate gland.
- *T3:* The cancer has penetrated the prostatic capsule and may have invaded the seminal vesicles. Two subcategories are further used. With *T3a* the prostate cancer has gone outside of the prostate capsule, but did not invade the seminal vesicles. *T3b:* The cancer has invaded the seminal vesicles.
- *T4:* With this tumor stage the cancer has grown into the tissues surrounding the prostate gland. This can involve the urethral sphincter, the bladder, the rectum or the pelvic tissues.

About the lymph nodes

The N categories describe whether the tumor has spread into nearby lymph nodes. *NX:* Lymph nodes nearby were not assessed. *N0:* the prostate cancer has not spread into nearby lymph nodes. *N1:* The cancer has spread to one or more local lymph nodes.

About metastases

The M categories describe whether the prostate cancer has traveled to distant parts of the body.

- *M0*: The cancer has not spread outside of local lymph nodes.
- *M1*: The cancer has spread beyond local lymph nodes. There are three subcategories.
- *M1a*: The cancer has spread to lymph nodes outside the pelvis.
- *M1b*: There is cancer spread to the bones.
- *M1c*: The cancer has spread to other organs like the lungs, the liver or the brain. There may or may not be bone metastases.

With all this information, the PSA values and the Gleason score from a prostate biopsy a new grid is computed as a stage grouping.

The Roman number classification is combined with the TNM classification as shown under this link.

http://www.cancer.org/cancer/prostatecancer/detailedguide/prostate-cancer-staging

For those who omitted the previous section, this passage will be of interest. It tells about survival rates of patients in the various stages of prostate cancer. Some men will find this prostate cancer risk calculator interesting:

http://deb.uthscsa.edu/URORiskCalc/Pages/uroriskcalc.jsp

The reason these staging classifications are important is because survival data correspond with each of the defined stages. This has been established through years of research and follow-up. The following table illustrates this.

Stage	5-year survival	10-year survival
I	100%	97%
II	89%	71%
III	80%	66%
IV	29%	0%

These numbers give you an idea of what kind of survival can be expected with various treatment options.

http://nethealthbook.com/cancer-overview/prostate-cancer/staging-prostate-cancer/

It is clear that the best long-term results can be achieved with stage I prostate cancer. This is a local tumor with no lymph gland involvement and no metastases. If PSA blood tests are regularly done and the doctor investigates when there is a rising PSA, most prostate cancer cases today should be found when they are in stage I. Stage II treated with ablation cryotherapy has a 10-year survival of 88% to 90%, which is significantly better than shown here. This likely is due to the cancer vaccination effect associated with cryotherapy that other methods do not have (discussed further in chapter 15). But other measures can improve the life expectancy, as is discussed in chapter 18 (Prevention of prostate cancer), for instance a balanced diet, certain supplements and the CaPLESS method (explained in chapter 15).

B) Genetic changes with prostate cancer

It is no secret that various genetic changes in a cell can cause uncontrolled cell division and spreading growth including metastases. This is also true in the case of prostate cancer. I like to keep it simple here and just review what we know at this point in time. But I will leave details about specific genetic loci out as they can become very confusing.

1. Family history of prostate cancer (hereditary prostate cancer)

The same gene BRCA2 that can cause breast cancer at a younger age in women has been shown to cause a testicle that is still in the abdominal wall because it did not descend into the scrotum (undescended testicle). BRCA2 can also cause Peyronie's disease where the penis is curved to one side when erected. The physician must be aware that there is a link between finding an undescended testicle in a boy or Peyronie's disease in a man and hereditary prostate cancer. These men need to have their PSA checked much earlier (perhaps starting at age 30 or 35) than men without a family history of prostate cancer.

http://www.harvardprostateknowledge.org/study-men-brca-gene-variant-psa-tests

Other tests have shown that there is a suppressor gene located on the long arm of the 13th chromosome of BRCA2 breast cancer patients. The same chromosome in males can cause familial prostate cancer when the suppressor gene is missing.

https://www.ncbi.nlm.nih.gov/pubmed/8909313

Twin studies have shown that the inherited risk for genetic prostate cancer is about 50%. Overall genetic studies did not detect only a few high impact genetic causes for inherited prostate cancer, but rather a larger number of low-impact genetic factors that have to come together like a perfect storm to produce inherited prostate cancer.

There are several other gene abnormalities located on different chromosomes that have been identified as causing inherited prostate cancer. Two of them involve normal immune system function. When these factors come together, there is inflammation in the immune system and defects in cancer suppression that initiate inherited prostate cancer.

2. Sporadic prostate cancer

This chapter is included to show, what genetic research is trying to accomplish. You may find the technicality of chromosome research too overwhelming! In this case you may want to skip over this very technical section. It is strictly included for completeness sakes!

When a man develops prostate cancer spontaneously without a history of prostate cancer in the family, it is called sporadic prostate cancer. A lot of research has been done with radical prostate cancer surgery specimens. Geneticists have analyzed these specimens and found that in 32% to 65% of prostate cancer cases the region p22 on chromosome 8 is often deleted. In patients with metastases, when lymph glands are examined genetically 65% to 100% have the same gene deletions on chromosome 8. Changes in the following chromosomes are often involved with sporadic prostate cancer: 6q, 7q, 8p, 10q, 13q, 16q, 17p, 17q, and 18q. There is no need to memorize anything of that complex genetic terminology. I am just mentioning it to show how complex the causation of prostate cancer is with interactions of multiple tumor suppressor genes located on several chromosomes. In aggressive end stage prostate cancer geneticists could show that hormone-refractory lymph node metastases were associated with changes in chromosome 8 at the q location. This was responsible for disease progression and resistance to hormone ablation therapy. On chromosome 7 a gene is located that is responsible for the production of caveolin. This is a prostate cancer-suppressing factor. When this gene is deleted or silenced by a near-by silencing gene, prostate cancer grows more aggressively or tends to metastasize earlier.

https://en.wikipedia.org/wiki/Caveolin

Tumor suppressor gene PTEN is located on chromo-some 10. It is often deleted in advanced prostate cancer cases. In one study 60% to 100% of advanced prostate cancer disease showed PTEN to have been deleted on chromosome 10 compared to localized prostate cancer where 0% of PTEN was deleted.

Loss of genetic material on chromosome 13 and 16 is associated with more aggressiveness of prostate cancer and higher probability of it to metastasize. Gene losses on chromosome 17 are rarely found in localized prostate cancer. This chromosome contains the important TP53 gene, which codes for a protein that regulates the cell cycle.

http://www.bioinformatics.org/p53/introduction.html

In advanced prostate cancer 40% were found to have a deletion of the TP53 gene explaining why the cancer cells divided rapidly in these advanced cases versus the slower growth in localized prostate cancer.

Deletions on chromosome 18 are mainly found in advanced prostate cancer cases.

One important gene for prostate cancer is located on the X chromosome (in the q11- q13 location) containing AR, which stands for androgen receptor. It is amplified in 30% of cases of advanced disease, which leads to failing hormonal ablation therapy. In contrast patients who have never been treated with androgen ablation do not show AR amplification.

At this point there are no rapid tests to screen for any of these genetic abnormalities associated with prostate cancer. But more modern sensitive tests to detect circulating nucleic acids (CAN) have been developed and are being used to correlate aggressive cancers with certain markers.

Reference: Wein, Alan J., MD, PhD(HON), FACS: "Campbell-Walsh Urology, Eleventh Edition", Copyright © 2016 by Elsevier, Inc. Chapter: Molecular Genetics and Cancer Biology.

3. Oncoblot test

One application from this type of research is the Oncoblot test.

http://oncoblotlabs.com/

Here the protein ENOX2 is measured in the blood. Normally this protein is only expressed during fetal life, but not in the adult. However, with 25 different cancers including prostate cancer ENOX2 is expressed again. As each cancer associated ENOX2 protein has a different isoelectric point, the exact cancer diagnosis can be given from this test. This allows a specialized laboratory to screen for different cancers, including prostate cancer.

I had this test done and it allowed me to clarify why I had a slowly rising PSA level; the Oncoblot test told me clearly that I was positive for prostate cancer, while the PSA level was equivocal at 3.0. While I was waiting for my mapping biopsy, the PSA level rose from 3.0 to 8.6. Three months after the cryotherapy was finished the PSA level went down to 0.9 and the Oncoblot test was negative. All these tests are useful to monitor the clinical situation of a prostate cancer patient. It also helps to determine that the treatment was successful.

4. Gleason score

We already pointed out that a higher Gleason score from a biopsy (let's say between 8 and 10) is due to a more aggressive prostate cancer than a prostate cancer with a lower Gleason score (Gleason 4 to 5). This histological information correlates with the number of genetic deletions and factors as explained under point 2 above that interact in making the cancer more aggressive. It may well be in the future that a cancer tests will become available where a print-out can tell which genetic factors are operative in a particular prostate cancer patient. But at this point all we have is the Oncoblot test, which is still rather expensive, and the PSA test, which is quite affordable. The Oncoblot test is specific and more sensitive than the PSA test. But the PSA test is still valuable as a screening test. The strength of the PSA test is when it is low. When it is high, we need to be aware that there can be all kinds of "noise" mixed in with the test. The values can be elevated with prostatitis, benign prostate hyperplasia and mechanical factors like riding a bike for a long time. All these various scenarios can elevate a PSA test, but they will not affect the Oncoblot test. The Oncoblot test just indicates whether you have or you do not have prostate cancer.

Conclusion

Staging of any cancer is important, because it deter-mines the prognosis of the outcome after treatment long before treatment has begun. The same is true for prostate cancer. The physician will need to know whether the cancer is just confined to the prostate gland as in stage I and stage II. It is important to explore whether lymphatic metastases or even distant metastases are present. This changes the survival rate from 97% in 10 years with stage I to 0% in 10 years with stage IV. As indicated the Gleason score gives information about the growth behavior, which also determines the long-term survival. Early detection is key to long-term survival. I have given a brief overview of genetics behind prostate cancer to give you an idea how complicated a disease this is. I showed you how this links to the results of biopsies with the Gleason score. I also introduced the Oncoblot test, a genetic test, which in my case was crucial to detect my own prostate cancer early. The PSA values were ambivalent, but the Oncoblot test was decisive.

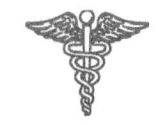

Chapter 5:

A Silent Killer

I'm Christina, and I work as a medical office assistant together with three other colleagues and two physicians in a suburban family practice.

This has been a busy morning, but now it is close to the noon hour, and the patient flow at the office is diminishing. Our team is not closing for lunch, but we are planning to take turns with our lunch break. The phone will ring, and we do not know, whether the call will be urgent or not. Often trouble strikes in the lunch break: it could be an accident of a child at school, a nosebleed, somebody who is out of a prescription, a skinned knee or something more critical, where the patient has to be sent to the emergency department. Often the events in a medical office are very much routine, but trouble also can strike without any warning.

This time the phone is quiet at noon, but instead the door opens and a man walks in, who seems to be a silent type. He rummages in his wallet and wordlessly takes out his medical insurance card. Jim Harrison, we read; he is fifty-six years old. No, he has never been a patient at this office, and so we start to prepare a chart for him. There are questions about his past health history, but not much information is forthcoming. He states that he has always been healthy, and at the question whether he has had any check ups in the past, he indifferently shrugs his shoulders. He does not believe in check ups, and he has not seen a doctor in twenty years. He does not have a family doctor either. Why should he bother? He is healthy!

We are looking at a tall man who looks strong and sturdy. The only thing that is noticeable is his posture; he is slightly stooped over. He volunteers that he has developed a persistent backache. It bothers him. His work is physically demanding, as he works in a lumber mill, but he denies that he got hurt at work. The backache just appeared, and he thought that maybe he had thrown his back out. He went to the drugstore and got some aspirin, but it did not really help. In the past month he saw a chiropractor, hoping that an adjustment would give him some relief, but it did not do the job. He denies that there are any other problems and goes to the waiting area. We all can see that he looks uncomfortable, as he walks with a slight limp. He grumbles about the wait, and when my colleague tells him that it will be a while, since he arrived without an appointment, his face becomes angry. He complains that he is wasting his lunch break. All he needs is some prescription to get rid of the pain, and for that he has to wait! Sullenly he sits down and grabs a magazine.

Patients who are unwell are not be the happiest individuals, and he is definitely miserable. We send the chart to the physician with a note attached, that this new patient is in pain and walked in without an appointment. As a result he is fitted in on an urgent basis, and after about fifteen minutes he sees the doctor, and a few minutes later he leaves rather in a hurry.

We are getting the chart back with the note of the physician: the patient was in a hurry, did not want a long discussion, but the doctor gave him a requisition for blood tests, a back x-ray and a small amount of pain killers.

One week later Jim is back, again without an appointment. This time he is not only miserable but also overtly hostile. This is a waste of his time! He has no time for doctor's office visits, and he has no time to be sick. And, by the way, the medication was entirely useless. His backache is still there, and if anything, it is even worse!

We notice the expression of frustration on the face of the doctor, when we retrieved the patient's chart. The patient picked up the prescription for painkillers, but he did not go to have the back x-ray, and he has not gone for lab tests either.

For two weeks we don't hear and we don't see anything of the patient with the sore back. In week three several sheets of test and x-ray results arrive from the laboratory and the x-ray office. We have to pass on all test results to the physician in a timely manner, and what we see on the results looks alarming: quite a number of the blood tests are abnormal, and the alkaline phosphatase is astronomically high. Even a medical office assistant knows that sky-high alkaline phosphatase levels are an indicator for trouble that is brewing in the bones! The x-ray result is like the last piece in a dark and ugly mosaic. The lower spine shows a large amount of lesions. The radiologist's report mentions that these lesions are compatible with widespread bone metastases. The doctor's face is somber. These are results that darken any day in a medical practice. One of us has to call the patient in. We cannot greet him with the most cheerful good morning voice, when we tell him that the doctor needs to speak to him about his test results. We also cannot tell him that the results are bad news. Making these kind of phone calls leaves us with a heavy heart, and a shadow hovers over the entire day.

We see the patient walk into the office, this time with an appointment. The doctor strongly suspects prostate cancer, and he sends his patient for more tests. Like with the previous appointments, this meeting with the doctor does not take long. The patient has no time for unnecessary appointments, and he has no time to be sick. Nothing has changed, except he now has the knowledge that he is facing an incurable and life threatening illness. If he is shocked by the verdict of the doctor, the stoic expression in his face does not give away any of the inner turmoil that he is very likely laboring with.

Within a week we see more test results, all of them ominous. The patient is terminally ill with prostate cancer and metastases. He is not showing up for a follow up appointment. We try to call him in, but there is no answer, when we call his home.

A report from the neighboring hospital explains more. This man, who lives alone, could no longer cope at home, and he had to be admitted to the hospital. Little can be done for him except palliative care to alleviate his pain.

It is never an easy day, when a report reaches the office, announcing that a patient has passed away. This particular report reached us only two months later. Jim has passed away in the palliative care unit of the neighboring hospital.

Yes, we are saddened and shocked. Cancer has once again reared its ugly head, and there was no help and no cure. The disease was only detected in its late stages and spread like a wildfire. Even three months of suffering are too much! All the statements that cancer can be cured or that cancer can be beaten sound like empty promises in a situation like that.

This was happening almost thirty years ago, and my co-workers and I wondered, whether we would live to see a time where prostate cancer would not remain a silent killer.

Conclusion

This was a case from my general practice 30 years ago. One of my colleagues treated this patient. We look back today and wonder what could be done differently now? At that time the only way to diagnose prostate cancer was by a rectal examination. But this patient did not see a doctor for 20 years; the cancer quietly grew and eventually metastasized into his bones. It was only then when my physician colleagues saw him. At that point it was an incurable cancer.

What could we do today?

The answer is that we should do yearly PSA tests from the age of 45 to 50 onwards. Once the PSA value raises, the doctor would refer the patient to an urologist for a prostate biopsy. The best form of biopsy, however is the mapping biopsy of Dr. Onik that delivers a complete histological picture of the prostate. Often prostate cancer is multifocal. There can be two, three or more foci of cancer. If this were the diagnosis from the mapping biopsy, the next step would be an ablation cryotherapy with or without the IRE surgery (more about this in chapter 15). This modern scenario has a much better prognosis. Early stage prostate cancer treated this way would have a 10-year survival rate of 96% to 100%.

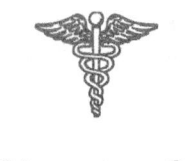

Chapter 6:

Help Comes Too Late

Fred has a way to light up the room with his big smile; he is such a pleasant humorous man, who is well liked by everybody. He is in his mid-seventies, and he is one of the regulars at the family practice where I work. The only alarm signals that come up in his health profile are his weight that is a bit too high, and as a result he now has high blood pressure. He does not smoke and he drinks only moderately. Old habits have stuck: he came to Canada as an immigrant from Germany, still loves sausages and beer, and the afternoon ritual of coffee and cake is firmly established. It is not the healthiest lifestyle, but we have dozens of patients who are similar: they show up at the office, have their blood pressure monitored, but otherwise they are hard of hearing when it comes to making some healthier life style choices or appropriate changes.

Otherwise Fred is quite diligent about appointments and compliant in taking his medicine. His blood pressure is controlled. He has not had a complete physical exam in two years, and the doctor suggested to him then that a rectal exam should be part of the general physical examination. He refused to have this done two years ago, and he is not too thrilled about this part of the examination now, like many men who also have a dislike for it. But this time he reluctantly agrees. The exam reveals that his prostate is enlarged, and it feels hard. This finding is abnormal, and he is referred to an urologist.

A relatively new test has recently become available, which is called PSA, short for prostate specific antigen. It is a simple blood test, and Fred is in agreement to have this lab test done before he sees the specialist. There are divided opinions in the medical community about the PSA test. It was first developed in the late 1970's, but only received FDA approval in 1986. Some health professionals shrug it away as a money-grabbing test and point out that it is unreliable. But other strong voices mention, that at this time it is the only screening test available for prostate cancer.

We are getting a lot of test results delivered every day, and Fred's PSA raises alarm flags. It is over 15, and with the finding of Fred's hardened prostate, it points to prostate cancer. The urologist suggests a biopsy of the prostate. It is an uncomfortable procedure, but the patient agrees to have it done. The pathology report confirms the diagnosis of prostate cancer. In view of Fred's age the urologist suggests radiation therapy rather than invasive surgery. Fred tolerates the radiation quite well. Life goes on, and for the next four years all seems to be well for him. The radiation must have been successful, and Fred and his wife are planning a celebration: they are happy to mark their fiftieth wedding anniversary! My husband and I are invited, but a month before the happy occasion Fred is seen at the office for some routine blood tests. Not everything is normal: the liver values have changed, and the PSA has shot up. The urologist sees the patient again in consultation, as the condition of the patient has very obviously turned unstable. The cancer is back, and it is very likely not only confined to the prostate. According to the blood test results the liver is affected as well. The specialist suggests a treatment with hormone inhibitors. The school of thought is that testosterone is the villain that fuels the growth of prostate cancer. In the past a removal of the testicles was another treatment, which was performed in the hope of stopping prostate cancer, which is an archaic and useless procedure. It deprives the patient of one of the pleasures he has left in life, the enjoyment of sex. Hormone inhibitors in the twentieth century are doing exactly the same. It is a bloodless but equally questionable treatment approach. Fred agrees to take the hormone inhibitors; he hopes that they will help.

Shortly before his Golden Wedding anniversary party more test results arrive at the office, and they do not look good at all. Normally it would be the proper procedure to call the patient in for the discussion of laboratory test results, but the doctor shakes his head. No, he cannot break this devastating news to his patient a few days before the celebration. Besides, the situation has turned from bad to worse, and nothing can be gained from discussing test results three days sooner rather than a few days later.

I still remember the party. It was a mood of thankfulness for fifty years of life shared together, but there was also a shadow of apprehension over the evening. I believe that Fred sensed that his illness had become worse. It did not destroy the celebration, but it definitely dampened the mood. I felt sad that this party would probably be the last one of togetherness for Fred and his wife, and it was very difficult for me to keep my sadness hidden; but it was a necessary thing to do. A few days later the doctor discussed the test results with Fred.

The urologist saw his patient in follow-up and referred Fred to the Cancer Control Agency, and the patient went in the hope that he could be helped. He came back for a lengthy conversation with his GP. The Cancer Control Agency had suggested a series of chemotherapy treatments, and this time Fred voiced his doubts. Now he was almost eighty years old, and he wanted to enjoy his days without additional suffering. He had seen relatives who received chemotherapy treatments that made them sick and miserable. Chemotherapy did not make any difference in their condition. It was like the beginning of the end. The cancer was not controlled, but wellbeing was destroyed and an already compromised immune system was dealt the final blow. He did not want to go the same way.

We understood his reasoning, and the doctor respected his decision. His GP made every effort to keep him at home where he felt at ease. Fred could not come to the office for appointments much longer, and so house calls were placed, when he needed pain control. He was suffering, and only strong pain relief was a measure to make his days more tolerable. Ultimately his liver failed due to metastases, and he sank into a coma. His suffering was over.

When a patient passes away, it is always a time of doubts and questions: what could have been done? What was missing to cure or to control the course of an illness? The sobering answer was very obvious: his disease was discovered too late. Screening tests in the early 1990's were only in their infancy. Radiation therapy extended his life by just a few years, and after that the disease returned with a vengeance.

It became painfully obvious that only early detection could help to cure a disease like cancer of the prostate. It also became very clear that hormone inhibitors are not an answer, but a crude and ineffective approach, and that radiation is not the cure either. And so the nagging question remained: which treatment is the best and the most successful one? Despite the fact that twentieth-century medicine has taken big steps forward in many areas of medicine, the treatment for cancer of the prostate still has a way to go till it can live up to the promise of a cure.

Conclusion

When I look back from 2017 I find it sad how I could not convince my patient to let me examine him two years earlier. But at that time the nerve-sparing highly selective prostatectomy was also not yet available. Unfortunately the radiotherapy treatment helped to slow down the cancer growth only for a few years. We now know that both radiotherapy and chemotherapy do not kill the cancer stem cells that are present with any cancer type. The end result is that the cancer comes back with a vengeance. Today patients with prostate cancer have more options to be treated. The best one today would be a mapping biopsy through the perineum to avoid infection and have a whole-gland biopsy. In the normal sized prostate it takes about 60 biopsy needles to map the cancer throughout the entire prostate. In a patient with BPH (benign prostate hypertrophy) this may involve 90 or even more biopsy needles. The specialist can then do an ablation cryotherapy, which has the best 10-year survival rate (100%). Cryoablation therapy destroys all of the cancer that was histologically identified. This method, pioneered by the interventional radiologist, Dr. Gary Onik will be discussed in more detail in chapter 15. With this method the cancer cells that have been killed also become the tool to stimulate the immune system in the sense of a vaccination against the patient's own cancer. None of these techniques were developed at the time, when my patient would have needed it.

But all of it is available now!

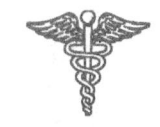

Chapter 7:

Stop the Hormones – But Does it Stop Cancer?

I studied medicine in Germany and have been a physician since 1971. A brief 3- year detour in cancer research at the Ontario Cancer Institute, Toronto/Ont. starting in October 1972 gave me some insights into basic cancer research. This was the place where stem cells were originally detected by Drs. James Till and Ernest McCulloch in the late 1960's. Our group was working on the same floor, but concentrated on the immune response to cancer. We were doing cell separations of different immune cells in a mouse model. I got tired of working in a mouse model as I wanted to study human cells, and so I left cancer research and re-entered into clinical medicine. I studied family medicine at McMaster University, Hamilton/Ont. for another 2 ½ years. Next I graduated with the Canadian State Exam (called LMCC) and started practicing family medicine in British Columbia in 1978.

The next 16 years I looked after many patients including also cancer patients. Since the late 1990's I became interested in anti-aging medicine. I became an A4M member (A4M stands for "American Anti-Aging Academy of Medicine"). This organization features a yearly world conference on Anti-Aging Medicine in Las Vegas, which I have been attending regularly since 2008. The reason this is relevant for the topic here is that Dr. Abraham Morgentaler, a Harvard trained urologist has given speeches on several of these conferences. His interest is testosterone and prostate cancer.

One of the driving hormones in a man is testosterone. It also is known that with age testosterone levels fall. The lesser-known fact is the importance of monitoring testosterone levels in aging males, so they have the choice of intervening with the aging process. Here are the facts about testosterone, about replacement of testosterone and about the anxieties of the medical profession to deal with this.

Androgen receptors contained in key tissues

Androgen receptors, https://en.wikipedia.org/wiki/Androgen_receptor are situated in the key organs like the brain, heart, muscles, bones, kidneys, fat cells, genitals, hair follicles and skin. They respond to all male hormones, called androgens, like testosterone, dihydrotestosterone (DHT) and DHEA. DHT is produced by metabolizing testosterone with the help of an enzyme, called 5alpha-reductase, http://www.medicalnewstoday.com/articles/68082.php in the adrenal glands. This is responsible for hair loss in males and some females. There is a genetic factor for this. It is important that the man continues to have all tissues stimulated by testosterone when he ages, or the key organs mentioned are going to suffer.

A lack of testosterone as the man ages (around 55 to 65) leads to a slowdown in thinking, osteoporosis in the bones, muscle atrophy (melting in of muscle tissue), and a lack of sex drive. The skin gets thinned and is more brittle. Mood swings can turn the male into the "grumpy old man".

Animal experiments have shown that the development of fatty streaks in blood vessels occur at a higher rate in castrated animals. The more encouraging finding in these animals is the fact that this condition is reversible by testosterone replacement. In healthy males of a younger age all organs are working well.

The problem starts when males age and the hormone regulation in the brain slows down, which ultimately leads to andropause in males, the equivalent of menopause in women. When testosterone is replaced in an aging man with low testosterone levels, the androgen receptors in key organs mentioned above are stimulated and normal organ function returns.

Reluctance of physicians to prescribe testosterone

It used to be taught to medical students that testosterone would be the cause for prostate cancer. This went back to an old observation by Dr. Huggins, a Canadian physician who practiced in Chicago. He took note that patients suffering from prostate cancer lived a bit longer after castration. The important detail that Dr. Huggins did not realize was the fact that testicles produce hormones, testosterone and small amounts of estrogen. When an orchiectomy was done because of the belief that testosterone production was the culprit inadvertently the real cause of prostate cancer, an estrogen surplus, was also removed. Due to the removal of the estrogen surplus the survival of these patients improved somewhat. Nowadays we have more sophisticated testing methods. Dr. Abraham Morgentaler (Ref. 1) has compiled a lot of evidence about the importance of testosterone in men. He proved, based on a lot more modern references, that it is not testosterone that is the cause of prostate cancer. We know now that estrogen dominance is responsible for prostate cancer and that this develops, as stated above, because of the low testosterone and low progesterone during the male menopause (also called "andropause"). Dr. Morgentaler, an urologist from Harvard University, has treated prostate cancer patients and put them on testosterone. To his and everyone else's surprise prostate cancer patients improved, their prostate cancer either disappeared or became much less aggressive, which can be measured by prostate biopsies with the Gleason score, https://wikipedia.org/wiki/Gleason_grading_system based on its microscopic appearance. The result was that they did better, not worse on testosterone!

Unfortunately the history of testosterone, orchiectomy and prostate cancer led to confusion among the medical profession. We now know that testosterone is innocent with respect to prostate cancer, testicular cancer or any other cancer.

But some of the old-timers among the physicians doggedly hold on to their false belief from the past because they were taught this way. If a man asks one of these physicians for testosterone replacement he may not only be told that he could not do that, but will also receive a tirade of false statements about testosterone.

We dealt with the myth of prostate cancer that is not related to testosterone treatment. There is another myth that older physicians often cite: that testosterone would supposedly be causing blood clots. At the University of Texas Medical Branch at Galveston (Texas, USA) a large study was done involving 30,572 men, ages 40 years and older. They all had venous thromboembolism and received an anticoagulant drug or an intravascular vena cava filter following their diagnosis. They also had a low testosterone level and were given testosterone replacement therapy. They were followed and monitored for further venous thromboembolism. None were found in any of the men.

The conclusion of the investigators was that filling a testosterone prescription was not associated with any clotting condition.

http://www.worldhealth.net/news/testosterone-therapy-no-link-blood-clot-disorders/

Aging and testosterone

The Massachusetts, http://www.ourstolenfuture.org/NewScience/reproduction/2006/2006-1210travisonetal.html Male Aging Study showed that testosterone has been declining in the male population over a period of 20 years.

Partially this was related to aging, but otherwise there may also be environmental factors, called estrogen-like substances or xenoestrogens, that have contributed to it as well. Although age is a factor, there is so much variation from man to man, that it is best to just measure testosterone levels and determine whether the total testosterone level is above or below 500 ng/dl (= 17.3 nmol/l). This seems to be the most reliable indicator in determining whether or not a man needs hormone replacement. The physician should also consider the risk factors that are the result of testosterone loss. These are: increased risks for prostate problems and/or cancer, cardiovascular disease, loss of bone density, a rise in cholesterol and urinary dysfunction. Dr. Randolph describes this in detail and also discusses who needs bioidentical testosterone replacement.

http://agelessandwellness.com/services-for-men/guide-to-mens-hormone-health

A New England Journal of Medicine study from September 2013 explained that apart from testosterone the male body needs a small amount of estradiol, the female hormone for normal functioning.

http://www.nejm.org/doi/full/10.1056/ NEJMoa1206168?que ry =featured_home&#t=articleDiscussion

This is achieved through the enzyme aromatase contained in fatty tissue. But testosterone replacement must be given as the bioidentical testosterone, so that a small amount of it can be converted by aromatase into estradiol. I have reviewed this in a blog entitled "The Full Story About Testosterone".

http://www.askdrray.com/the-full-story-about-testosterone/

Risk of prostate cancer

Having reviewed the hard facts about prostate cancer risk, it is now clear that older men get prostate cancer because of lowered testosterone in their blood and increased body weight, where fat converts androgens by the enzyme aromatase into estradiol; this leads to estrogen dominance. Estrogen dominance causes breast cancer and uterine cancer in women and prostate cancer in men. When the total testosterone level in a man is lower than 500 ng/dl (= 17.3 nmol/l), it is a sign that he needs testosterone replacement therapy to protect his prostate from prostate cancer. Additionally, replacement of testosterone in older men does not cause prostate cancer, but rather improves the outlook of prostate cancer patients when testosterone is given to them.

I am fully aware that these new insights will be news to a lot of physicians, including urologists and also to prostate cancer patients.

Conventional teachings regarding hormone therapy

Conventional medicine uses hormone therapy:
1. When prostate cancer has spread too far to be treated with surgery or radiation.
2. When prostate cancer comes back after surgery or radiation has failed.
3. Along with radiation therapy, if your cancer is aggressive as based on a high Gleason score, the cancer is outside the prostate capsule and your PSA values are very high.
4. Before radiation therapy to make the tumor shrink, which makes the radiation more effective.

The methods used to do hormone therapy are orchiectomy (surgical castration) or luteinizing hormone-releasing hormone (LHRH) agonists. This is also known as GnRH agonists. These drugs shut down the production of testosterone in the testicles and they are very expensive.

Conclusion

Hormone therapy in prostate cancer is a confusing topic, because the reasoning of conventional medicine is completely contrary to the truth. As Dr. Morgentaler has shown, testosterone treatment is safe and does not cause prostate cancer or make prostate cancer worse. To the contrary, the worst prostate cancers are found in the group of men who have the lowest testosterone blood levels.

Treatment of these men with testosterone improves their histological Gleason score! The key is early diagnosis by doing regular PSA levels. If this is found to be rising above 20 or 30, have a timely mapping biopsy done to locate the prostate cancer. The next step is to treat it with ablation cryotherapy to eradicate all cancer as explained in chapter 15.

If your testosterone level is low, replace what is missing with bioidentical testosterone creams or testosterone injections. This will prevent an early death from a heart attack or stroke. Men have testosterone receptors for a reason. I do not believe in crippling a man with prostate cancer using the barbaric hormone ablation methods discussed. Why make a eunuch out of a male cancer patient? This is absurd. If there is testosterone deficiency, replace it!

Ref.1: Dr. Abraham Morgentaler: "Testosterone for Life – recharge your vitality, sex drive, and overall health" McGraw-Hill, 2009

More information:
https://www.cancer.org/cancer/prostate-cancer/treating.html

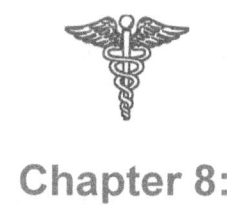

Chapter 8:

Active Surveillance for "A Little Bit of Cancer"

As I mentioned in the introduction, there is no safe waiting or active surveillance with regard to any cancer. Cancer cells make it their business to grow. They don't wait to see what you are going to do. In the case of prostate cancer they simply fill the space surrounded by a tough prostatic capsule. When this capsule is full, the cancer cells have enzymes that enable them to break though the barrier and invade the surrounding tissue. They also find the lymphatic drainage and spread into the surrounding pelvic lymph glands. In addition they can invade the blood vessels and metastasize to other areas of the body like the lungs, liver, brain or bone.

The urologist does not really know what your type of prostate cancer will do. It is not prudent to lull yourself into the belief that it is safe to sit back because you only have "a little bit of cancer" that is confined within the prostate gland. It would rather make sense for the urologist or your general practitioner to order a testosterone level as we discussed in chapter 7. If your testosterone level is low, chances are high that your Gleason 6 prostate cancer could grow into a more aggressive Gleason 7 or 8 type cancer.

A good 2014 review of "active surveillance" can be found under this reference:

https://www.ncbi.nlm.nih.gov/pmc/articles/PMC4144844/

One of the tools to decide whether or not a patient with prostate cancer is a good candidate for active surveillance, is the use of multiparametric magnetic resonance imaging (mMRI). This special MRI scan can distinguish between a more aggressive form of prostate cancer or an indolent prostate cancer.

Another tool is to use the PSA density, where the PSA value is divided by the prostatic volume.

https://www.ncbi.nlm.nih.gov/pmc/articles/PMC4565896/

When these additional criteria are used for classifying a patient as being suitable for active surveillance, the reclassification during future biopsy results because of worsening Gleason scores is only 4% in patients where mMRI and PSA density was used versus 20% to 30% when these criteria were not used (Campbell- Walsh "Urology", Eleventh Edition, Copyright © 2016 by Elsevier, Inc.).

Not every center that offers active surveillance uses mMRI's and PSA density. As a result their assessment of who should go for active surveillance will not be that accurate. A reclassification at a later date following a follow-up biopsy is more likely.

Criteria of active surveillance

The reviewers made the point that the majority of prostate cancer patients do not need a radical prostatectomy, as this procedure has significant complication rates. The following criteria were used to include a person for active surveillance.

- Gleason score equal to or less than 6
- PSA value equal to or less than 10ng/ml
- Stage T1 up to stageT2a
- Less than 2 biopsies with less than 50% of prostate cancer involvement in each biopsy
- Some studies had an age cut-off point of 70 years or older. But the authors discuss that younger patients as low as 60 years of age and older could also be included, particularly when they are well educated and motivated.
- Statistics have shown that less than 6% of patients older than 65 die from their diagnosed prostate cancer, if not treated with radical prostatectomy or radiotherapy and if their Gleason score is less than 7. In order to avoid a break-through of prostate cancer, active surveillance has to be done in a responsible way. This includes:
- PSA and prostate palpation (rectal exam) every 3 months for 2 years; twice per year thereafter
- Follow-up biopsy 1 year after the initial biopsy, then every two years
- The trigger for a change to active intervention is when low risk changes to intermediate risk or high risk, based on Gleason score, PSA or prostate cancer stage

Statistics regarding active surveillance

One of the cautions based on the research by Dr. Gary Onik, as we will see later, is that typically those patients who have been followed with active surveillance are frequently one stage worse than assessed by the methods just mentioned.

Dr. Onik does mapping biopsies, which are whole prostate perineal biopsies (one biopsy needle every 5 mm) so the entire prostate is scanned by biopsies for prostate cancer. This results in a histological map of the location of the prostate cancer within the prostate gland. In a normal sized prostate this involves 60 needles, in an enlarged prostate it can involve 90 needles, all done under a general anesthetic. In the routine transrectal biopsies no more than 20 biopsy needles are used, which leaves lots of room for errors. The rectal biopsy needles are also blind whereas with the mapping biopsy every needle is kept track of geographically through a grid system.

9% of patients are getting anxious and may request a change from active surveillance to active intervention. A Baltimore study (John Hopkins) involving 769 men is cited in the above mentioned 2014 review. 81% of the men were free of intervention after 2 years, 59% of the men after 5 years and 41% of the men after 10 years. After 2.2 years on average 255 men (33.2%) underwent intervention. Of these men 188 (73.7%) were undergoing intervention on the basis of disease reclassification after their biopsy.

A Danish study found that after 5 years of active surveillance 60% could continue to stay on the program while others had been reclassified to active intervention. In a study that involved 9,557 patients with organ-confined disease and a Gleason score of 6 or less only three patients died of prostate cancer. The 15- year mortality risk to die from prostate cancer was only 1 percent.

http://www.uptodate.com/contents/active-surveillance-for-men-with-low-risk-clinically-localized-prostate-cancer

There seems to be a place for highly reliable and compliant patients with early prostate cancer that satisfies the above-mentioned criteria to go on an active surveillance program. The key is to have an open mind and be willing to switch at any point in time to an active intervention program.

One point to be cognizant of is that even MRI scans can err, as will be mentioned below. It may come as a surprise, but MRI's are not infallible. Even an MRI scan may only show one lesion in one lobe of the prostate, whereas a high sensitivity Doppler ultrasound may show several separate lesions in both lobes of the prostate. This immediately changes the stage of the prostate cancer.

Here is a good, detailed overview of how active surveillance works in a retired man who has been diagnosed with prostate cancer:

http://www.harvardprostateknowledge.org/choosing-and-sticking-with-active-surveillance-a-patients-story

Active Holistic Surveillance

Dr. Katz, an urologist and integrative physician is using an "active holistic surveillance" for patients with uncomplicated early prostate cancer. The thinking is that you have been advised to do active surveillance for an early prostate cancer that does not require treatment at the present time. You might as well do something to improve your health in general, which will also benefit your prostate cancer. As a result you likely won't need as many biopsies. You do require PSA tests every three months and you require a repeat MRI scan every year. But if there is no change, you won't need a biopsy at that point in time, which differs from the regular approach of active surveillance.

http://www.ascopost.com/issues/february-25-2016/active-holistic-surveillance-may-prevent-unnecessary-biopsies-in-low-and-lowintermediate-risk-prostate-cancer/

As this link explains, the patient eliminates red meat and increases instead the intake of fish or poultry. There is an increase of fresh vegetables like kale, broccoli, spinach and cauliflower. One to two tablespoons of freshly ground flaxseed is added to oatmeal or yogurt every day. Dairy intake is reduced except for organic yogurt. Refined sugar intake is reduced. Cow's milk is replaced by soymilk. Instead of white pasta whole-wheat pasta is recommended. One to two cups of green tea should be consumed every day, as well as one glass of red wine with dinner two to three times a week. Patients also make liberal use of pomegranate juice, vitamin D3, vitamin E, selenium, lycopene and the multi-herb anti-inflammatory formula called Zyflamend. This contains ten herbs with antioxidant and anticancer action.

In a study examining the active holistic surveillance over 40 months only 12% of the patients dropped out. 88% continued with the program. Patients often did not require a further biopsy, as the yearly MRI test and the three-monthly PSA test were stable. The key here is to continue your regular check-ups with your doctor or urologist, so that you do not miss a sudden activation of your prostate cancer. Don't get carried away and think you will never get a biopsy again or that you are safe from needing other procedures done.

Radical prostatectomy versus active surveillance

PSA screening has led to earlier detection of prostate cancer. As a result biopsies are done more often and when prostate cancer is found, radical prostatectomies tend to be done fairly liberally. This has led to some unnecessary surgeries. A study conducted at the Cleveland Clinic showed that of 179 men who underwent radical prostatectomy (removal of the prostate and more) between 2004 and 2008, about 71% would not have needed the surgery. Furthermore, many of these patients are now impotent and incontinent.

Unfortunately, some developed other serious, long-term side effects from the surgery and in about 30% of them the cancer returned. Here is a detailed review article that lists all of the side effects of radical prostatectomy.

https://www.ncbi.nlm.nih.gov/pmc/articles/PMC3922321/

The bottom line is that one should be cautious and think about all of the findings carefully. Depending on the age of the patient and the findings, active surveillance may be indicated instead. If the Gleason score, the PSA finding and the rectal examination deteriorate, this would be the time to intervene. But it may be a mapping biopsy followed by ablation cryotherapy rather than a radical prostatectomy that would be the preferred method of surgery. Cryotherapy has a much lower complication rate than a radical prostatectomy in terms of urinary incontinence, rectal incontinence and erectile dysfunction. It also has a recurrence rate of only 6% in 10 years (versus 30% recurrence for radical prostatectomy).

Conclusion about active surveillance

Sweden and Denmark have reliable cancer registries. They followed prostate cancer patients and found that there were high rates of prostate cancer deaths among those men who postponed treatment. For men below the age of 75 who were diagnosed with non-metastatic prostate cancer, there was a greater than 50 % chance of dying of prostate cancer, if they did not receive immediate treatment.

On the other hand a study from Quebec City showed that there was a 69% reduction in prostate cancer deaths in those men who were screened for prostate cancer and were immediately treated.

Overall it is clear that watchful waiting (also called active surveillance) is not a good option. Delay in treating any cancer is bad news for the patient; this applies to prostate cancer as well!

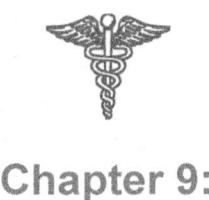

Chapter 9:

Detected in Time

I have seen a change to my career; I'm no longer working as a medical office assistant in a medical practice, but my interest in medicine has not diminished. With the arrival of the twenty-first century a lot more information about health and lifestyle has emerged. Anti-aging medicine is becoming a force, and new tests and scans are giving more insight into the function of our bodies. The Internet has long become a source of information to the public. As a result we are no longer satisfied with the information that we are receiving during a short appointment with a doctor. We are asking more questions and have become more proactive and vigilant. But one thing has remained the same: we are confronted with health or the lack of it in our daily lives as much as in the past.

This year has been tough. My mother just passed away, and even though she lived to be to one hundred, the death of a close family member is always difficult to cope with.

A phone call today does not make the day any brighter. A close family member is calling, and he described that he has seen his GP for a checkup and test results. The one alarming piece of news is a high PSA. This screening test for prostate cancer has become accepted as a screening tool over the last ten years. He also mentioned that he is scheduled for an appointment with an urologist. He does not sound too anxious and is pretty pragmatic: it is just something that has to be done. My husband and I wish him all the best, and after a week we are informed that our relative is scheduled for a prostate biopsy. It is another step to find out whether there is cancer and at what stage it is.

We are confident that this procedure is the best way for the specialist to design a treatment protocol, but a few days later our world is shaken up by another phone call. His wife is very distraught: her husband had the biopsy and went home. He received some antibiotics to avoid a possible infection after the biopsy. A few days later he collapsed at home and had to be taken by ambulance to the emergency department of the hospital. He has a raging fever, and the diagnosis is infection. It was casually mentioned to him this could occur as a side effect to the biopsy, and unfortunately this was the case in him. It does not stop there.

While he is in the hospital the infection escalates, and he develops septicemia. The condition is grave, he spends two weeks in hospital between life and death, and only after the administration of three different antibiotics does he gradually recover. This was a close call!

We are shocked and wonder how this could ever happen. Here is a diagnostic test that is supposed to help with a life saving treatment, but the test almost killed the patient! The explanation is very logical: the biopsy of the prostate is done through the rectum of the patient. Even a layperson knows that the rectum is not the cleanest area of the body.

It teems with an army of bacteria, such as E. coli. Since the biopsy needle punctures the rectum, these nasty bugs can freely migrate into the blood of the patient, and once they are there they will multiply.

This can even happen, when the patient receives some antibiotics to prevent infection. If the numbers are large and they are migrating through the entire bloodstream, septicemia is the next step, and E. coli infections can kill.

We are relieved for our relative that this hurdle is over. A diagnosis has been achieved, and now there is the uncomfortable knowledge that he indeed has prostate cancer.

He announces that he is going to have a consultation with his general practitioner. We are hopeful, but what we are hearing next shakes our confidence. The general practitioner is not too concerned about the cancer. He states that it is "low grade" only. He makes it sound like a minor annoyance that does not need much attention: the buzzword is "watchful waiting" (now called "active surveillance"). Next he predicts that his patient would very likely not die of the disease, as he is already seventy-five years old. He is not concerned about the risk of prostate cancer and mentions that he would probably die of a heart attack, a stroke or old age first!

Next he sees the urologist. Since he is rubberstamped as being "old", the specialist is talking about possible radiotherapy, which he considers to be the "proper" approach. We are appalled at this verdict! Our relative has always been healthy, does not have cardiovascular disease and comes across as younger than his age. We are fully aware that radiotherapy will give him a few years only, after which the disease will return, as not all the cancer cells have been killed by radiation. The remaining cells will be resistant to radiotherapy and create a firestorm of metastatic disease within a few years. It sounds like bad medicine that does nothing to cure a disease, even though it has been detected early enough!

I personally also wonder about the definition of low-grade prostate cancer and the approach of "watchful waiting". How sensible is it that we are watching a small problem and wait till it gets big? Cancer is a fact. There is no such thing as a "little bit of cancer"! It is like making an insane statement to a woman that she is "a little bit pregnant!" Except there is a fine difference: at the end of a pregnancy is new life; at the end of cancer is death!

We are getting another progress report from our relative after he discussed his condition with his GP next. He reads the consultation report and is satisfied with the opinion of his urologist colleague. When his patient wonders about surgery, the doctor smiles and explains the treatment plan like a benevolent uncle who tries to explain proper conduct to a wayward and not too bright nephew. In his opinion surgery is unnecessary. Why would a seventy-five year old undergo a fairly invasive surgical procedure? Radiation is perfectly adequate and very effective!

I know that he will not get into a verbal fight with his long-term family physician, but I also know that he has questions, when we receive a phone call from him. He wants to talk to Ray.

I'm Ray, and I just had a conversation with my relative.

I explained to him what I learnt long time ago when I did cancer research for 3 years. We had to participate in lectures on radiation physics and the professor explained to us that with any radiation therapy there is a cancer survival curve that is followed. On that curve you kill a certain amount of logs of cells off. But by definition there will always be a few cancer cells left. You cannot kill the last cancer cell off with radiotherapy as this would kill the patient's immune system as well. You are limited with the total dosage of radiotherapy, and at the end of radiotherapy a few cancer cells are remaining that have become radio resistant. These may sit there for a long time, but after a few years they multiply, and next we have a cancer patient with a vicious radio resistant cancer. I also explained to him that I had attended a continuing education lecture from an urologist in Vancouver, BC. He stated that early prostate cancer should not be allowed to spread, but should be treated with a suprapubic radical prostatectomy. I explained this to him and told him also that the urologist from Vancouver did not say that there was a "cut-off" for prostatectomy at a certain age.

He agreed to a referral to this urologist surgeon, and I arranged for this. Faithfully he went back to his family physician to report that he was not having radiotherapy. He wanted a second opinion by a specialist who was an experienced surgeon. If he had wanted a non-confrontational talk with his GP, he was in for a surprise. The good uncle of the previous appointment had vanished and turned into an angry man! Instead of a listening ear he now got a tongue lashing from the doctor, who was not pleased about a patient asking inconvenient questions and questioning medical treatments. A less self-assertive patient could have been intimidated by this behavior, but he ignored the tirade and saw the other specialist. The specialist explained to him that there are some differences between the two treatment approaches. He mentioned that radiotherapy was the treatment that gave a "five-year guarantee", but with the surgery he would have at least a "ten-year guarantee." This logic was enough for the patient to decide for surgical treatment. He had to take a medication to shrink the prostate, and a few months later the procedure was done at a Vancouver hospital.

Conclusion

Radical prostatectomy is the "gold standard" in treatment for prostate cancer in the early 2000's. A new approach is to preserve the nerves, and it is a procedure that is very intricate and done with the help of a microscope. Nowadays the robotic prostatectomy has miniaturized the tools to do the same surgical procedure. When it is all done, the patient should be free of prostate cancer, and his sexual function has been preserved due to the fact that every effort was made to not injure the nerves to the penis.

Our relative is one of the success stories, as his cancer is gone. He never had a recurrence. Despite the crystal-ball predictions of the physician that he would die of a stroke, a heart attack or old age, he is active, alive and well at the age of eighty-nine, fourteen years after the surgery. This is even better than the "ten-year guarantee." It has to be mentioned that not everybody is so lucky. According to a Johns Hopkins study the laparoscopic prostatectomy has a 10-year survival rate of only 77%. There is a high rate of cancer recurrence (up to 20 to 30%), if not all the areas of prostate cancer have been removed. Doctors have called prostate cancer a "multifocal disease", which means that there may not just be one area of the prostate that is affected by cancer, but there can be more areas affected with prostate cancer. Having a "radical prostatectomy" does not mean that all the prostatic tissue is removed. As a result, the remaining tissue can still harbor cancer, which was not detected at the time of the surgery. This can be the cause of cancer recurrence after what appeared initially to be a "successful" surgery.

In the beginning of the twenty-first century we are still left with the uncomfortable question, what can be called "successful". It is true: big steps have been made to screen for prostate cancer earlier than was the case 20 years ago. On the other hand a rectal biopsy is risky business. Surgery techniques have become more intricate to remove cancer, but it is still an early diagnosis that makes the surgery less invasive with less side effects.

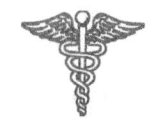

Chapter 10

Radical Prostatectomy a Success?

Radical prostatectomy is a surgical procedure that has been developed to remove early prostate cancer when it is still confined to the prostate gland within the capsule. There are three main approaches.

1. One is to open the lower abdomen with a vertical cut from the belly button to the pubic bone. A second horizontal cut in the pubic area joins the vertical cut to make the total incision look like an inverted T. This allows the surgeon maximal visualization when the wound edges are opened up. The surgeon digs into the pelvis below the bladder to locate the prostate gland. This is an approach from the top down. This was the surgery that was used in our relative's case. In this procedure the surgeon can take samples of lymph glands and send them for histology. The bigger the tumor is, the more likely that the neurovascular bundle may have to be cut as the tumor is removed. There are two of those bundles, one on each side. Cutting into this area can lead to erection problems, although, if one neurovascular bundle is

untouched, erections can re-occur within 1 year from the surgery. With this procedure a lot of cutting was done behind the pubic bone and below the bladder. It is not surprising that patients complain of a lot of pain.

2. A second approach is to go upwards from below. The surgeon enters through the perineum, the space between the back part of the scrotum and in front of the anal opening. With this perineal approach a curved line that crosses the perineum is used to open the space from below. Often the nerves that control erections are cut with this approach, which causes erection problems. This surgery is faster than the retro pubic one and less painful, but the patient may later regret having signed the consent when erections are lost.

3. In recent years urologists have miniaturized radical prostatectomy by introducing laparoscopic methods to do prostate surgery. This started with laparoscopic radical prostatectomy (LRP). Here the surgeon introduces long specialized instruments through several small incisions. A light source is also introduced allowing the surgeon to see everything in detail on a video camera. There is less bleeding, faster postsurgical recovery and less pain following the surgery. The da Vinci method or robotic prostatectomy is just another variation of the laparoscopic prostatectomy with the same outcome.

More details about any type of radical prostatectomy

Here is a brief description of what steps are involved in any of the radical prostate surgeries: radical prostatectomy, suprapubic radical prostatectomy, laparoscopic radical prostatectomy or robot-assisted laparoscopic radical prostatectomy. This is based on Ref. 1 and 3 (at the end of this chapter).

- For staging purposes the lymph nodes around the pelvic veins are removed for pathological examination.
- The dorsal vein in front of the prostate gland is tied and cut to diminish the risk for bleeding.
- The urethra, the tube between the bladder and the outside is severed to allow the surgeon better access to the prostate.
- The neurovascular bundle is identified and preserved as this contains the pelvic nerves supplying the corpora cavernosa, which is necessary for penile erection.
- Division of the bladder neck is next for improved maneuverability of the prostate.
- Resection of the seminal vesicles is performed (prostate cancer often affects the seminal vesicles).
- Resection of most of the prostate containing the prostate cancer is next.
- Construction of a urethrovesical anastomosis is the final step. (The divided urethra and bladder have to be repaired at the end of the prostate surgery).

Risks and side effects of any radical prostatectomy

Generally speaking, the earlier a diagnosis of prostate cancer is made, the smaller the cancer is. If surgery is done by any of the methods described, there is a lower risk to damage the neurovascular bundle on each side of the prostate. When the tumor is bigger, extending to the outer reaches of the prostate close to the neurovascular bundles, it is likely that the surgeon has to remove one or both bundles. This means a loss of sexual function, which most men fear.

Generally speaking those men who have a life expectancy of more than 10 years benefit from radical prostatectomy most. The older he is, the less likely he will benefit from a radical prostatectomy.

You can see this from these figures:

- 3 patients out of 4 (75%) had surgery at ages 56 to 65 years
- 2 in 5 (40%) had surgery at ages 66 to75
- 1 to 2 in 10 (10% - 20%) had surgery at age >75 years

What are some of the risks of radical prostatectomy?

There is the risk of the anesthetic. This is why the physician will want to do an EKG of the heart to check the rhythm and perfusion of the heart. If there is any abnormality, a referral to a cardiologist will be made to ensure it is safe to do a general anesthetic. There can be bleeding during the surgery and also some bleeding through the urine after the surgery. Every man who has this type of surgery will be left with an indwelling catheter for 1 to 2 weeks. This can cause an infection in the bladder and the urethra, which may have to be treated with antibiotics. Like with any general anesthetic there can be blood clots in the legs that may dislodge and travel into the lungs as pulmonary emboli. These have to be treated with blood thinners. There can be damage to nearby organs like the bladder neck or the urethra. As mentioned, if the cancer extends to include the neurovascular bundle, this has to be excised, which won't allow the patient to have erections any more.

On rare occasions a bowel loop may be injured, which happens more with laparoscopic and robotic surgery than with open prostatectomies. If this happens, the surgeon has to do bowel surgery to prevent abdominal infection. When lymph nodes are removed, there can be an accumulation of lymph fluid (a lymphocele), which may have to be drained.

Direct side effects of the prostate surgery

Side effects are urinary incontinence, erectile dys-function, shorter penis size and risk of inguinal hernia.

There are quite a few problems that can be encountered during this type of surgery. Blood vessels that are cut can bleed. When cautery is used to take care of bleeders, there is a risk that the electric current damages the nerves in the neurovascular bundle. There is an effort made by some surgeons to use mini vascular clips instead to avoid this from happening. The ureter, the tube coming from the kidney and going into the bladder, can get injured. The rectum in the back can get perforated. If so, there are a lot of E. coli bacteria in the rectum and this could contaminate the wound and even lead to septicemia.

Complications after prostatectomy surgery

Following the surgery there can be clots developing in the deep leg veins. They can get dislodged and migrate into the lungs giving the patient extreme shortness of breath. Blood thinners may be required for a few months. There can be a leak in the urethrovesical anastomosis, the area where the urethra has been repaired. In this case further surgery to repair the leak is needed. There can be postoperative bleeding. The patient will have an indwelling catheter from the bladder to the outside. A certain amount of blood in the urine is normal for a few days. As the blood is diluted with urine, the red urine looks worse than it is as very little blood can stain the urine red.

The death rate from a prostatectomy (within 30 to 60 days) lies between 0.4% to 1.6%. This depends on the age of the patient and other contributing diseases.

Urinary incontinence

There may be leakage of urine or dribbling. This may normalize in time, or it may not, particularly if the bladder neck was injured when removing prostate cancer from the upper part of the prostate gland. Stress incontinence is the most common form of incontinence following prostate surgery. Here the man leaks urine when he coughs, laughs, sneezes, or exercises. It stems from a partial damage to the bladder sphincter that forms the valve between bladder and urethra. Overflow incontinence occurs when there is scarring of the bladder outlet. This leads to trouble emptying the bladder. It takes a long time to urinate and there is very little force behind the stream causing dribbling of the urine. Another form of incontinence is urge incontinence. Here the bladder is oversensitive to stretching, so the patient feels the urge to urinate, even when fairly little urine has accumulated. After a few weeks of healing this type of oversensitivity usually stops.

Following prostate surgery normal bladder control usually returns after several weeks to a few months. Older men usually have more incontinence problems than younger men. Larger cancer centers, where surgeons do a lot of surgery and are very experienced, tend to have fewer complications than in facilities, where this surgery is not regularly performed.

The indwelling urinary catheter stays in place for 1 to 2 weeks. This allows the vesicourethral anastomosis to heal. However, when the catheter is removed, there often is urinary incontinence due to a lax sphincter muscle. Physicians call this an "intrinsic sphincter deficiency". What this means for the patient is that urine leaks at all possible and impossible occasions, a real annoyance. Patients were followed for two years and asked then what incontinence rate they had.

92% to 98% had no leakage of urine at that time meaning that between 2% and 8% still had urinary incontinence.

Erectile dysfunction

When a man does not have sufficient erection to be able to have sexual penetration, he is said to have erectile dysfunction or impotence. This is very common following prostate surgery. Often there is an injury to one or both of the nerves going through the neurovascular bundle and becoming the cavernous nerves that go to the corporal bodies of the penis. In many cases when the tumor has reached a bigger size and has invaded the neurovascular bundle the surgeons must remove the cancer along with the structures of the neurovascular bundle to save the patient's life. But this leads to severe problems with erections. When no neurovascular bundle was injured during surgery the man will likely recover his full sexual function within 3 to 6 months.

For 4 to 6 weeks he needs to heal and will not feel like sex. From then on he needs some help with medication for erectile dysfunction.

Sildenafil (Viagra), vardenafil (Levitra), and tadalafil (Cialis) are the commonly known pills that are used for this purpose. Side effects from these drugs are headaches, flushing, upset stomach, light sensitivity, and a stuffy or runny nose.

With Cialis 6 to 8% of patients develop excruciating lower back pain. They seem to be more sensitive to this medication, but halving the dose or taking the 5 mg tablet only every second day may solve the problem (avoiding back pain, but having erections).

It is getting more complicated for men where both neurovascular bundles were cut. A vacuum pump can be used to create an erection. The pump is placed over the penis. As the air is sucked out by the pump, blood is drawn into the penis.

The erection is maintained by a strong rubber band that is placed over the penis base after the pump has been removed. After sex the rubber band is removed. If other methods do not help, a penile implant can be considered next. This has to be surgically placed inside the penis. There are several devices that are available.

At 2 years following radical prostatectomy patients complained about their sex life as follows: 56% complained of poor erections, 42% of difficulties with orgasm, 64% that erections were not firm and 53% of poor sexual function.

(Cited by: Niederhuber, John E., MD: "Abeloff's Clinical Oncology" Copyright © 2014 by Churchill Livingstone)

Shorter penis

In a radical prostatectomy where a short piece of the urethra is removed along with the prostate, the overall penis length can become shorter. This becomes noticeable with the erected penis when compared to the length prior to surgery.

Risk of inguinal hernia

A radical prostatectomy increases the risk of getting a future inguinal hernia in the groin area.

10-year survival

As mentioned already according to a Johns Hopkins study the laparoscopic prostatectomy has a 10-year survival rate of only 77%. This does not compare favorably with Dr. Onik's ablation cryotherapy with a 10-year survival rate of 100%.

15-year survival study

Abeloff's Clinical Oncology cites a publication by Eggener et al. 2011, which followed 11,521 men for cancer-specific survival after radical prostatectomy for prostate cancer. The cumulative prostate cancer deaths at 15 years were only 7%. The main predictors of whether the survival was good or bad was the Gleason score, the presence or absence of seminal vesicle invasion and lymph node metastasis. Here are the specific mortality rates:

Gleason score dependent survival

15 year prostate cancer mortality of 0.2% to 1.2%: Gleason score of 6 or less
15 year prostate cancer mortality of 4.2% to 6.5%: Gleason score of 3+4
15 year prostate cancer mortality of 6.6% to 11%: Gleason score 4+3
15 year prostate cancer mortality of 26% to 37%: Gleason score 8 to 10

Localized versus invasive cancer

15 year prostate cancer mortality of 0.8% to 1.5%: organ-confined cancer
15 year prostate cancer mortality of 2.9% to 10%: extraprostatic extension
15 year prostate cancer mortality of 15% to 27%: seminal vesicle invasion
15 year prostate cancer mortality of 22% to 30%: lymph node metastasis present

This study aptly shows how important it is to detect prostate cancer early. It also shows how important it is to remove it early to get the best long-term survival. In my opinion the statistics also speak against the concept of doing active surveillance, as the tumor will just slowly increase in size and spread.

Conclusion

There are limits with respect to the success rates of radical prostatectomy. All of the various techniques like conventional prostatectomy, laparoscopic prostatectomy and robotic prostatectomy lead to the same statistics of long-term survival rates. We have now 15-year survival data split into Gleason score based survival. We even have 15-year survival data based on whether the prostate cancer initially was local or had spread. Prostate cancer with a lower Gleason score has a better survival than prostate cancer with a higher Gleason score.

But one factor has not been examined with regard to the long-term outcome of radical prostatectomies. There is a difference between a mapping biopsy and the standard transrectal prostate biopsy. A mapping biopsy consists of at least 60 biopsies that represent the histology of the entire prostate gland. Random transrectal biopsies leave big gaps where cancer may be hiding, but the treating physician does not know. This difference may well explain the discrepancy between the better survival with ablation cryotherapy and the gold standard radical prostatectomy.

More information:

1. Niederhuber, John E., MD: "Abeloff's Clinical Oncology" Copyright © 2014 by Churchill Livingstone
2. Eggener SE, Scardino PT, Walsh PC, et al: Predicting 15-year prostate cancer specific mortality after radical prostatectomy. J Urol 2011; 185: pp.869-875
3. https://www.cancer.org/cancer/prostate-cancer/treating.html

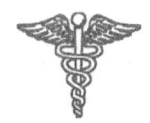

Chapter 11:

The Robotic Revolution

In the previous chapter we discussed the radical prostatectomy including the laparoscopic resection of the prostate (LRP). A newer variation of this method is the robotic prostatectomy. Don't worry, there are no robots doing the surgery. It is still the surgeon who is in charge. But he/she uses a robotic interface, called the "da Vinci system", which the surgeon controls sitting at a control panel (the console) in the operating room.

The crazy thing is that everybody thinks because it is high-tech it would be better or superior to any of the other methods. The truth is far from that.

The advantage of this system is that the instruments are easier to maneuver and move more precisely than with the original LRP. The overall outcome is the same as with the open procedures or the LRP. And no matter, which technique is used, the outcome still depends on the skill of the surgeon!

But here is what the urology text indicated below points out:

- A three-dimensional, multi-level magnification spec-trum is built into the surgeon's console
- The one-centimeter thin robotic arms and the da Vinci system's sensitive electronics make the surgery a lot more precise than traditional laparoscopic methods
- This means that robotic surgery removes cancer tissue with an ease and precision unheard of before
- The surgeon will not harm healthy tissue as much, which allows for less scarring and allows for a much shorter recovery after surgery

The FDA cleared the da Vinci Surgical System in 2000 for adult and pediatric use for multiple applications including prostate surgeries.

Despite all of these advantages robotic prostatectomy remains just another form of total prostatectomy with the same dangers to the neurovascular bundles resulting in potential erectile dysfunction and problems with bladder control.

Here is what a textbook says regarding robotic assisted radical prostatectomy: "Damage to the nerve bundle can occur because of direct incision, entrapment in a suture or clip, thermal injury, or traction" (Campbell-Walsh Urology, Eleventh Edition, Copyright © 2016 by Elsevier).

An alternative, which is a less invasive procedure, would be ablation cryotherapy. I will explain this in detail in chapter 15.

Medical help with erections following prostate surgery

If the cancer was found early and did not involve the neurovascular bundles on each side of the prostate, there is hope that the surgeon who does a robotic prostatectomy will be able to save the nerve connections. When the surgeon has to use electro cautery to stop arteries from bleeding or if the cancer has grown into the neurovascular bundle and this has to be removed, the probability of regaining sexual potency may be seriously delayed.

http://www.urology.uci.edu/prostate/potency.html

This link shows that potency can take 18 to 36 months to come back following robotic prostate cancer surgery. 41% of men who were younger than 65 years were operated with robotic prostate surgery using the electro cautery free technique. They had their potency back within 3 months.

If nerves were spared on one side, 35% of those above 65 had their potency back by two years after the prostate surgery. If both nerves had to be cut because of cancer involvement, only 13% had their potency back after 2 years. When both neurovascular bundles could be saved, 43% of men had their potency back 2 years after the prostatectomy surgery.

Between the times from 4 weeks after prostate surgery to whenever that magic recovery (spontaneous sex) takes place, there is a period where medical help is needed. Pills like sildenafil (Viagra) and tadalafil (Cialis) must come to the rescue. Taking Viagra 50 mg or 100 mg daily and Cialis 5 mg every other day can help to get your "sexual rehabilitation done". The magic seems to happen when the two pills work together every other day. But every man is different, and you need to talk to your own doctor whether these pills are right for you and what dosage you should use.

Mortality rates following robotic prostate surgery

As already mentioned earlier the Johns Hopkins study using laparoscopic prostatectomy has a 10-year survival rate of only 77%. Despite the high-tech approach there is no improvement over these survival figures with the robotic prostatectomy, because this type of surgery is based on incomplete pathological data from random rectal biopsies. Now there is a new study from the New York University Langone Medical Center, New York, NY. Date Oct. 2015.

https://www.ncbi.nlm.nih.gov/pubmed/26163812

This study, which involved a cohort of 1864 men stratified risks based on postoperative Gleason scores. Three risk categories were identified: low risk (Gleason 4-6), intermediate risk (Gleason 7) and high risk (Gleason 8-10). After 10 years of follow-up the survival was 99.2% for low risk prostate cancer, 99.0% for the medium risk group and 88.5% for the high-risk group. Overall these are excellent survival statistics, which emphasizes how important it is for a good long-term survival to do PSA testing regularly and immediately go to a treatment center when the PSA is rising. If you miss that point you will only reach a lower survival rate.

Another study from Switzerland that was released in August 2016 was done on 100 patients with stage 2 and stage 3 prostate cancers. 79% had stage 2 disease, 15% stage 3 disease. Following laparoscopic prostatectomy the 10-year cancer specific survival was 98% and the overall survival was 93%.

https://www.ncbi.nlm.nih.gov/pubmed/26710661

If you want to improve the 10-year survival rates with any kind of procedure to treat prostate cancer, you need to consider Dr. Onik's mapping biopsy. As I will explain in detail in chapter 15, a mapping biopsy is a grid-like biopsy done under general anesthetic where 60 to 90 biopsy needles are placed every 5 mm until the entire prostate has been mapped. The biopsy samples are sent in separate tubes, carefully labeled, to the pathologist for histological analysis. With this baseline it is clear where the cancer is situated geographically within the prostate. Using this knowledge the cancer can be eradicated using cryosurgical ablation.

Conclusion

Statements like "I had surgery with the da Vinci system" or "I had robotic prostate surgery" may sound mysterious, but despite the technical advance this does not make it a superior method. The Vancouver General Hospital in Vancouver, BC ran a trial published in 2014 to show that the results with the robotic prostatectomy technology were identical to the conventional, open prostatectomy.

https://www.ncbi.nlm.nih.gov/pmc/articles/PMC4001645/

As long as urologists do rectal biopsies on a hit and miss basis, nothing will change in the long-term statistics. The conventional method is missing cancer, and it is from these missed areas that recurrences originate. With a mapping biopsy all of the cancer that was detected is removed, which improves the long- term survival statistics.

More info:
http://www.roboticoncology.com/robotic-prostate-urgery/

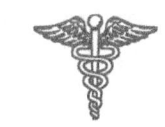

Chapter 12:

Radiation, Brachytherapy & Proton Therapy

There are three major radiation therapies of note, conventional radiation therapy, brachytherapy and proton radiotherapy. I will deal with each of them in sequence.

Radiation therapy

Radiation beam therapy has been used for several decades and has been improved technically to reduce the effect on the healthy surrounding tissue and increase the curative effect on prostate cancer.

There is a new study where patients were followed for 11 years that compared the effects of only hormone ablation therapy with a combination of hormone ablation therapy and radiation beam therapy. The survival of men receiving the hormone ablation therapy alone was 77%. The combination therapy (hormone ablation and radiotherapy) had an 11-year survival of 90%.

http://www.cancer.net/fewer-men-dying-prostate-cancer-
10-and-15-years-after-combined-treatment-radiation-
therapy-and-anti

The downfall of radiation therapy are urinary incontinence problems, erectile dysfunction that can be permanent
and bowel problems from radiation to the rectum. But the
overall long-term survival statistics of radiation therapy is
more successful than brachytherapy or proton therapy.

Radiotherapists have developed modified ways to apply
radiotherapy, attempting to deliver the radiation to where
the cancer is, but minimizing the side effects on the urinary
tract, the bladder and the rectum. Intensity-modulated
radiation therapy delivers the radiation to geometrically
complex fields. If you combine this with imaging techniques
you get image-guided radiation therapy. This allows the
intensity-modulated radiation therapy to be aligned with
the target area. The bottom line is better delivery of the
radiation where it should be delivered to, but fewer side
effects.

Radiation side effects

The main damage of radiotherapy is to the microscopic
blood vessels of the bladder, the lining of the rectum, the
sphincter muscle of the bladder and the urethra. About 33%
of radiotherapy treated patients develop rectal irritation
(proctitis) or bladder irritation (cystitis) during the course of
radiotherapy. In the majority of cases this settles following
completion of the radiotherapy treatment. But 5% to 10%
are left with permanent symptoms. These patients develop
irritable bowel syndrome or intermittent rectal bleeding.
They may also have bladder irritability and intermittent
blood in their urine. Intensity-modulated radiation therapy
was found to have less rectal irritation than other forms

of radiation therapy (like proton therapy or 3D conformal radiotherapy). External beam radiotherapy causes more damage to the rectum than to the bladder and urethra, compared to brachytherapy.

Long-term effects of radiotherapy

There are different cell populations within the prostate gland; some are radiosensitive, but others are fairly resistant. One study looked at this and found that within the fields of radiation there were up to 40% of radiation resistant cancer cells in the center of the prostate cancer. In another study a group of prostate cancer patients was radiated with a high dose of radiation and 2 ½ years later repeat prostate biopsies were done. Surprisingly almost 50% of patients had still the original prostate cancer present. All these biopsy positive patients have a poor long term prognosis. Surgery usually fails at the margins (when not all cancer is removed), radiotherapy fails in the center of the tumor where not all cancer is killed by radiotherapy.

Another problem with radiotherapy is long term development of new radiation-induced cancers. This often happens in the rectum, the bladder and the urethra. These are all sensitive tissues that develop DNA breaks and new tumors develop over the decades. Researchers found this particularly when more than 10 or 20 years had lapsed since the date of the radiation treatment.

Ref.: Campbell-Walsh Urology, Eleventh Edition, chapter "Radiation therapy" © 2016 by Elsevier

Brachytherapy, the new buzzword

Medical approaches to various illnesses have pro-gressed. "Life extension" and "anti-aging" have become new buzzwords over the last ten years. Our human condi-tion has not changed.

It is 2009 and we just had a chat with a neighbor. He is concerned, as his PSA test is quite elevated. In the meantime the tug-of-war about the PSA test for prostate screening has settled down a bit. After all, this is really the only screening test available for prostate cancer! There are still voices that say "no", but vigilant males are saying "yes". It is not a deterrent that in some countries the medical insurance does not pay for this test, and it is the patient who has to foot the bill. The price is between 25 to 40 dollars for a PSA test, but there is the additional fee for a doctor's visit. Nevertheless, it is better to be safe than sorry!

John is at the end of his sixties, and apart from the disturbing test result he is healthy. The most appropriate approach at this stage will be a referral to a urologist. He will need a biopsy. It is not a pleasant procedure, as the patient will experience severe discomfort due to the fact that the local anesthetic will not block all the pain. There is also the ominous risk of infection with the transrectal approach.

We are talking to John a month later. He had his biopsy, and it is indeed positive for prostate cancer. Luckily he did not have infection to deal with. He has received the advice of the specialist that brachytherapy would be the best treatment modality for him. It has been explained to him that the insertion of radioactive seeds into the prostate to kill the tumor is much less invasive than a radical prostatectomy. It sounds easy: a radioactive substance is inserted under anesthesia, and it only kills the cancer cells nearby, but other areas of the body are not affected. This certainly sounds less menacing than radiation therapy. He is very much in favor to go ahead with this procedure. After all, radical prostatectomy has a much longer recovery time. He is also concerned that after surgery erectile dysfunction is very common, and he does not want to undergo surgery for this reason. Many men think exactly like him!

Although I understood what his concerns were, I explained to him that radiotherapy could only kill a certain proportion of his prostate cancer cells. The ones that are left will regroup and become more vicious as resistant prostate cancer cells. As he had an early cancer, I felt that like with our relative, a total prostatectomy would be the wiser choice, giving him a better chance for long-term survival. He disagreed and went for the brachytherapy.

What is brachytherapy?

With this form of radiotherapy radioactive seeds the size of rice grains are introduced into the prostate with needles. Depending on the size of the prostate the radiotherapist places 70 to 150 of these needles through the perineum skin (between the scrotum and the anal opening) into the prostate. This is done under spinal anesthesia or general anesthesia. Transrectal ultrasound (TRUS) is used to control the deposit of the radioactive seeds into the right spots. The radioactive seeds with iodine-125 or palladium-103 are deposited into the prostate before the needles are withdrawn. Iodine-125 has a half-life of 59.4 days; palladium-103 has a half-life of 17 days. The radiation is not reaching very far, but it is irritating enough that sometimes a radiation proctitis can develop in the rectum. This causes rectal pain and may also lead to diarrhea for a period of time. Other complications are urinary problems with incontinence. This develops a few weeks after the treatment, but the condition will gradually improve. Erection problems are another complication, but these problems are somewhat less prominent than following a radical prostatectomy. Younger patients do better than older ones.

The seeds stay in place. Because of the short half-life of the isotopes the radiation fades away after a few months.

After the implant has been completed, usually a CT scan is done to check the post implant location of the seeds. When a patient has a large prostate due to benign prostatic hyperplasia, the prostate has to be pretreated for 6 month with androgen suppression therapy. This will shrink the prostate to a normal size, which makes the placement of the radioactive seeds much easier.

For intermediate risk patients where the cancer is still local there have been excellent 5-year survivals of 85%. The 7-year survivals were reported to be 80%. Another study showed less than 6% PSA recurrence in low or intermediate risk patients over a 10-year follow-up period.

Urinary symptoms are more common following brachytherapy, more so than after external beam radiotherapy. Urinary blockage occurs in 22% of patients.

However, a small surgery ("channel transurethral resection") can restore voiding function while continence is preserved. Erectile function is preserved in 62% to 86% of patients who were treated with brachytherapy alone. These figures are lowered when external beam radiotherapy is combined with brachytherapy. But Sildenafil (Viagra), vardenafil (Levitra), or tadalafil (Cialis) can be used alone or in combination to overcome erectile dysfunction.

Ref.: Campbell-Walsh Urology, Eleventh Edition, chapter "Management of Localized Prostate Cancer" © 2016 by Elsevier

2016 John is back

As John had moved away, we had no contact with him for 7 years. But our paths crossed again when he moved back, and we met him by chance. He had back pains due to metastases to his lower spine. He also had some metastases in his pelvis, as he was told. He had spot radiation treatments with external beam radiotherapy. But he mentioned that his PSA levels were still going into the

400 ranges. This is a sign that the tumor was disseminated and was growing out of control. The cancer center suggested giving him chemotherapy to control the cancer better. But after only one treatment he developed a flu-like illness with skyrocketing temperatures. He ended up in hospital for several days and was treated with antibiotics. His blood tests were also out of line. A blood transfusion perked him up again. After this experience he felt that he did not want any more chemotherapy or radiotherapy. Here we are looking at a man in the end stage of prostate cancer. He had put his hope into brachytherapy, but it could not solve the cancer problem for the reasons I mentioned above: only a certain percentage of cancer cells gets killed, the rest come back and are resistant to chemotherapy or radiotherapy. Chemotherapy is not much different: most cancer cells are knocked off, but a small percentage of them will survive and return as chemotherapy resistant cells. Eventually nothing works anymore, and the patient dies. This was true also in John's case. He died in early 2017.

This example should serve as a deterrent to any man, who hears that brachytherapy is an effective treatment or offers a cure. At the same time it is painfully obvious that chemotherapy at its worst is making the patient sick and only pretends to control a condition before it leads to the demise of the patient. Studies have been done with patients when radiotherapy or brachytherapy has lost its effectiveness. Often the oncologist will suggest hormone ablation therapy, which sometimes responds for a few years. But if this stops working the oncologist likely will suggest the use of a mix of chemotherapeutic agents that may add a few month to the patients life, however rarely more than one year.

http://www.uptodate.com/contents/chemotherapy-in-castration-resistant-prostate-cancer?source=see_link

What conventional medicine does not tell you

You may wonder why a 70 year-old patient is immediately referred for brachytherapy rather than a prostate surgical treatment. First, there is the implied thinking that radiotherapy calms the cancer down for at least a few years and that the aging patient will likely die of another medical condition. Secondly, there is a dark side to organized medicine that is difficult to understand. I heard that a urologist makes about 5,000 $ for a radical prostatectomy. If a brachytherapy treatment costs 22,000 $ there is lots of room to give the referring urologist a kickback fee, which may or may not be higher than the surgical fee. Nobody wants to talk openly about the exact kickback habits that are in place. This will also change from state to state and country to country. But I find this a dangerous situation when clinical judgment is clouded by financial incentives rather than by the objective need of the patient. This disturbing unethical practice is kept under wraps, but it only reinforces, how cancer is big business at the expense of the patient! Here is a website that mentions some cases in the U.S.A.

http://www.derivativesinvesting.net/article/364962556/c-r-bard-settles-allegations-of-kickbacks-to-promote-radiation-treatment-for-prostate-cancer/

Comparison of brachytherapy and total prostatectomy

A 10-year follow-up study at Johns Hopkins following a radical prostatectomy, which excluded men with positive lymph nodes, indicated that 77% had PSA levels less than 0.2. The authors considered this a cure.

http://urology.jhu.edu/newsletter/prostate_cancer56.php

The Georgia Center for Prostate Cancer Research, used brachytherapy plus external-beam radiotherapy to treat prostate cancer. Between 1984 and 1993 men in this series had an open retro pubic implantation of radioactive seeds.

At 10 years, the Georgia Center reported that 57 % had a PSA of less than 0.2. The Hopkins results indicated that 77 % of patients who had a radical prostatectomy during the same time period had PSA levels less than 0.2. That's a difference of 20 percent! There is another study that quoted a 72% 10-year survival with brachytherapy alone.

https://www.moffitt.org/File%20Library/Main%20Nav/ Research%20and%20Clinical%20Trials/Cancer%20 Control%20Journal/v8n2/163.pdf

In that study the 5-year PSA-negative survival was 79% and 75% of cancer recurrences occurred within 5 years.

This means that brachytherapy's success rate for treating prostate cancer is much worse than radical prostatectomy (20% worse!). If we take the better values of 72% at 10 years, brachytherapy is still 5% worse than radical prostatectomy. But the concerning factor is that 75% of recurrences happen in the first 5 years. This is what happened to Jack!

Be cautious when you listen to different urologists and surgeons. When you judge which method to treat prostate cancer is best, use the procedure that has the highest survival numbers at 10-years. This is how the quality of a treatment program is measured. The next step is to assess the side effects that are associated with the treatment procedure.

The Pacific Northwest Cancer Foundation in Seattle, WA reported that 5.1 % of patients were incontinent, and 1.7 % of men had such severe incontinence that they needed a urinary diversion done. This is an attachment of a bag that is worn under the clothes to be able to collect urine.

Compare this to Dr. Onik's ablation cryotherapy: his 10-year biochemical disease free survival for intermediate stage prostate cancer was 89%. For early stage prostate cancer there was a 10-year survival rate of 100% with 94% being disease-free and 6% having recurrence of cancer (measured by elevated PSA values). This is 11% better for intermediate prostate cancer than the Johns Hopkins study and 17% better for early prostate cancer than the Georgia Center study. Urological complications were negligible; there were no long-term potency issues after 3 to 5 months.

http://www.prostatecancer2.com/attachments/File/ Long-Term_Results_of_Optimized_Focal_Therapy_for_ Prostate_Cancer.pdf

Proton radiation therapy

Protons are atomic sub particles that can be used instead of traditional beam radiation. They get through the healthy tissue without doing much damage (contrary to radiation). When they hit the prostate cancer they explode and release their energy, which is where the damage should occur. Proton beams can be used to treat cancer. As explained they cause less damage to surrounding healthy tissues.

But before patients can be treated you need to have access to an accelerator (cyclotron or synchrotron) that creates the proton particles. You also need a transport system to carry the beam from the accelerator to the patient. Finally you have to have a delivery system to control and shape the beam to the three-dimensional configuration, which can deliver it to the tumor site in the patient.

1. The University of Florida Proton Therapy Institute did a 5-year prospective follow-up study.

http://www.proton-therapy.org/prostate_cancer_study_21114.html

Investigators reported that the cancer-free 5-year survival for low and intermediate risk were 99%, while for the high-risk patients it was 76%. Gastrointestinal complications were 1.4%, the urinary complication rate was 5.3%.

2. A 10-year follow-up study was done by the Loma Linda University Medical Center in a group of 1255 prostate cancer patients. They were all treated by proton therapy. The overall disease-free 10-year survival rate was 73%. Low risk patients with an initial PSA of less than 4 had a 10-year survival rate of 90%.

https://protonbob.com/sites/default/files/files/!Ten%20Year%20Study.pdf

The combined gastrointestinal and genitourinary toxicity was 6.6%.

There is only one flaw and this is the cost. It takes a lot of expensive equipment to generate protons that can be used for proton therapy. Because of this there are only a few institutions in the US that offer proton therapy. On the other hand, there are many radiation clinics all over the US offering regular radiotherapy treatments. Given the good survival statistics in combination with hormone ablation therapy regular radiation therapy would be preferable in my opinion over proton radiation therapy and/or brachytherapy. You heard what happened to John who had brachytherapy. He developed multiple metastases in the bones and died in the beginning of 2017.

A case of radical prostate cancer surgery followed by radiation therapy

I know Art as a happy and upbeat older man, who has lived in the neighborhood for a long time. It is rare that he complains, and he enjoys golfing in summer, goes bowling with his buddies, loves his glass of wine, and he loves a chat with the neighbors and a good joke.

We crossed paths back in 2005, when my husband and I went for a walk in the neighborhood, and he was working in his yard. When he saw us pass by, he stopped his work. It was a signal that he was in the mood for a chat. We expected a funny story or one of his jokes, but this time was different. He knows that my husband is a physician, and he wanted to talk about a health problem. This is nothing new for us. It happens frequently that a friend or neighbor wants to bounce ideas around about health, life style or health problems.

Art mentions that he has had a check up with his family doctor one month ago. Over the past few years the values of his PSA test have been creeping up on him. First he was not too worried about it, but after a rectal exam his physician was concerned, as he has found an enlarged prostate. Recently Art has been sent to an urologist. The specialist told Art that he needed a prostate biopsy fairly soon. Now Art wants to know, how soon he should go for this procedure. He is definitely not looking forward to it, as he has been informed of the possible side effects of infection. Ray explains to him that he should not procrastinate. This is about his health, it is about getting a diagnosis, and you simply don't play games with your health by postponing an important test. Our neighbor is satisfied with this information. He cracks a joke that the biopsy would keep a few people off the unemployment row, such as the nurse, the doctor and the hospital receptionist, and he agrees that he will have the biopsy done soon.

A few weeks later we are on one of our evening walks again, and our neighbor flags us down. He reports that he had the biopsy with the comment "Man, that was a bitch". It was painful, but luckily he did not get an infection. He grimaces as he mentions that the results were positive for prostate cancer. The urologist has told him that he has the choice of a surgical procedure called "radical prostatectomy" or an approach with brachytherapy. Art looks at us and doubtfully shakes his head: "Brachy- what the hell! I don't trust this new-fangled stuff!" He mentions that he believes that cancer should be cut out and thrown in the garbage. He is a man who believes in a practical approach, as he points to the diseased branch of one of his apple trees: "See this? This is sick, and it has to come off. I'll take the saw to it. You don't do brachy-something!" He uses farmer's wisdom: if there is a bad growth in the body of a human, surgery should take care of it. He wants it gone and is determined to have surgery!

It turns out that Art is getting his surgery within two months. We wish him luck before he is going in for the procedure. We see him, when he is back at his place, and he is still convalescing. He mentioned that the doctor told him that the tumor seemed to be fairly large, but he thought that he got it all with the surgery. We see our neighbor puttering in his yard about a month later, and we wonder how he is doing. We notice that some of his spunk is no longer there. He is relieved that he is at home, but golfing is not on the agenda, bending down to pick up a bowling ball is painful, and he has to take it easy with garden work. He mentions that it hurts to wear regular pants, and he wears sweat pants instead, as they don't put pressure on the area.

Demonstratively he lowers the pants to show his scar. We are not surprised that he still has pain.

We are happy for him, when he reports that after two months he is finally pain free. However, not all is well for him. For a while he had to wear an indwelling catheter, which has been removed. He expected that everything would be back to normal after that, but with an embarrassed expression in his face he confides that he has constant urine leakage. He went back to the doctor to mention this problem, but he received the rather negative news that this is due to an injury of his bladder neck during surgery. This is a known complication, and he needs to live with it, and he was told to use incontinence garments from the drugstore. The doctor mentioned to him that in some patients rectal leakage could also be a problem. This is not a source of comfort to our neighbor, and he states that adult diapers are no fun! He wants to stay young, but not this young! He cracks a joke about another problem: "You know what? Sex is now a word from a foreign language dictionary!" Dejectedly he shrugs his shoulders, as he adds that he has been warned about erectile dysfunction after the surgery. He is disappointed when he mentions: "It is all crap! Those little blue pills are not doing their job either. Life is not the same after surgery." There is only one positive item left, which is as important for him as for his wife of forty years. The cancer is gone after the surgery. There are negative consequences, but he is alive; not alive and well yet, but alive!

As time goes on Art seems to be back to his old self. He mentions that he had to adjust to changes in his life. He is no longer embarrassed to wear incontinence garments. It is a necessary evil, which is due to the surgery. And what about sex? He acknowledges that he had his good times in the past. He looks over to his wife with a grateful smile: "We may not have sex, but we still have each other."

For five years nothing untoward happens. Art is still living in the same neighborhood. By now he is in his late seventies, but he has kept busy and has been well. One day we see worry in his face. We stop and wonder, what is going on. He mentions that he has had regular check ups, and out of the blue his PSA level has jumped up, when it was just a bit elevated before. He is rightfully concerned that his prostate cancer could be back. His doctor has already made a referral for him to see an urologist. We try to encourage him. He sounds frustrated, when he states: "I just can't see myself go through hell again like five years ago." My husband tells him that he will very likely receive a different treatment. There will be no surgery. He sounds somewhat relieved, but all the same he is afraid: "Life has been good, but I don't feel like dying. It would be nice to hang around here a bit longer!"

We hear that our neighbor is going for tests. One of them is an MRI scan. The verdict is not entirely surprising; there is a recurrence of cancer. He is told that there are some lymph nodes that are affected in the area. It is unfortunate, but he is lucky that the cancer is not in his bones. The next step will be radiation therapy. He expresses his worry, when he talks about the upcoming radiation treatments: "I heard that this radiation stuff can make people really sick. What if I pee all the time and sit on the toilet all day with diarrhea? That's worse than a dog's life!" My husband tries to calm his concerns and explains that not everybody has severe side effects.

After several weeks the treatment has been completed. We see Art busy in his usual fashion. He is working outside again and is talking to a few neighbors recounting his last few weeks. The sense of gloom is no longer there. He reports that despite retirement his last few weeks were like going to work again five days a week for regular radiation treatment. No, it was not bad! He had no pain, and there was not much trouble with side effects. He sounds optimistic. "Let's hope that this will be the end of it." We wished him the best!

In the meantime five years have passed. Art is still part of the neighborhood. He has been a fighter through surgery and its side effects. Five years after the initial surgery he faced radiation therapy for a recurrence, and he went through it. Of course he has been aging, but his old spunk is back. He is still chatting with the neighbors and cracks jokes, goes golfing and bowling, and he is happy to report that he knows from his doctor that his PSA levels are close to negative. They have been low and stable like this since his radiotherapy treatment. There is no recurrence of the disease, and he states: "I'm a lucky man! Every day above the ground is a good day." He is eighty-three now. May he enjoy more years in good health.

Conclusion

The problem with all forms of radiotherapy is as follows:

1. Radiotherapy will only kill a certain amount of logs of the cancer cells. There will always be a tiny percentage of cancer cells that are left behind. When the radiotherapy treatment is finished these cells will regrow, but they also will be radiotherapy resistant, which makes the cancer recurrence much more difficult to treat. But there are exceptions like Art's case.
2. There are prostate cancer stem cells that can cause regrowth of prostate cancer. I will explain in chapter 15 in detail that prostate cancer stem cells survive radiotherapy treatment unharmed, which is the reason why cancer cells regrow from them about 4 to 5 years from the date of the radiotherapy treatment.

3. All radiation therapy, except proton radiation therapy to a lesser degree, leaves collateral damage in the surrounding normal cells. This causes a lot of side effects from the ionizing radiation including new cancers just at the time when the patient hopes to be healed.

The way to measure the overall effectiveness of a certain type of treatment is to determine the 10-year survival data. For brachytherapy this 10-year survival is 57% as explained before. Standard radiotherapy combined with hormone ablation therapy had an 11-year survival of 90%. The Loma Linda University Medical Center had an overall disease-free 10-year survival rate of 73% for proton radiotherapy. Low risk patients with an initial PSA of less than 4 had a 10- year survival rate of 90% for proton radiotherapy.

Based on this proton therapy, which is much more expensive than the other radiotherapy treatment modalities has the best survival rates at 10 years among the radiotherapy treatment modalities.

But when you compare this to ablation cryotherapy, this has the highest survival rate of 100% at the 10-year follow-up point. 94% of the patients treated with ablation cryotherapy were completely free from any recurring prostate cancer.

This is based on low PSA values with the follow-up at 10 years. 6% of patients had recurrent prostate cancer, which could be treated again with cryotherapy. Compared to all of the radiotherapy options ablation cryotherapy is the better treatment option. I will discuss this more in chapter 15. Before I go there I like to review whether lasers can do anything for you.

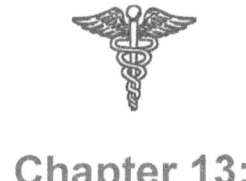

Chapter 13

Intervention with Laser - The Light of Hope?

Laser applications have entered the world of medicine some time ago.

At higher energy you probably know that lasers can be used to remove small unsightly veins or flat warts. But laser is not only used for cosmetic procedures. These higher energies can also be used to do laser ablation prostate surgery. Low-dose laser phototherapy is a newer procedure that has originally been used to treat lung cancer and esophageal cancer. It is being tested to treat prostate cancer as well.

Blue laser guided prostate laser ablation

This treatment modality involves the depiction of the prostate tumor on an MRI scan. This information is creating a 3 D geographical map of where the tumor is located. Subsequently the MRI guides a blue laser ray to the focus where the tumor is located, and the high-energy laser eradicates the tumor. The advantage is that the application is very precise. If the tumor is early and is situated far enough away from the neurovascular bundle, this is good news for the patient's sex life and bladder control in the future. Another advantage is that the procedure can be repeated anytime in the future, should there be a recurrence.

More info:
http://sperlingprostatecenter.com/focal-laser-ablation-new-york-city/?ibp-adgroup=adwords&gclid=Cjw KEAjw7svABRCi_KPzoPr53QoSJAABSvxfVIVV-fvwRHIO5SfaUv50fA8wT8lvUii2FRLmKNdLQRoCS6rw_wcB

Laser ablation therapy

Laser ablation therapy under MRI guidance is a newer procedure for prostate cancer that is still considered experimental by the insurance company Aetna:

http://www.aetna.com/cpb/medical/data/800_899/0843.html

In this medical overview it is pointed out that there are no long-term studies comparing this treatment modality to other established treatment modalities. There are efforts to standardize MRI guided laser ablation therapy for prostate cancer.

https://www.ncbi.nlm.nih.gov/pmc/articles/PMC4080850/

At this point there is no consensus what would be the best way to do laser ablation. At the present time recruiting is going on in the US for a laser ablation trial, but no 10-year survival rates using this procedure are available at this time.

https://clinicaltrials.gov/ct2/show/NCT02759744

It goes without saying that at this point I would not recommend such an experimental procedure. You need to know what the 10-year survival rates are!

Low-dose laser phototherapy

Phototherapy is a new type of treatment where cancers are destroyed using low-dose laser beams that activate a chemical substance that is taken up in the cancer first. Normal cells absorb the photosensitizer also, but they eliminate it while it stays around longer in cancer cells. Common radio sensitizers are Chlorin E6, Hypericin and Curcumin that are activated by different laser light frequencies. This low-dose laser phototherapy has been successfully applied in people with lung cancer and esophageal cancer. The reason there are some limits is due to the fact that laser beams penetrate tissues only to a certain degree. This can be overcome with a new infrared laser that is penetrating tissue up to a 5 cm depth. Three frequencies are employed with the Weber system that correspond to the absorption peaks of the three photosensitizers, red light (658 nm) to activate Chlorin E6, yellow light (589 nm) to activate Hypericin and blue light (405 nm) to activate Curcumin.

http://www.dr-weber-laser-clinic.com/en/the-laser-therapy/the-principle/

If a plastic catheter is inserted through the prostate into the bladder, the treating physician can insert a laser applicator and place it into the center of the prostate gland. When an appropriate photosensitizer is given intravenously before the laser treatment, which matches the laser light frequency, this can be used to treat prostate cancer.

The problem with this treatment modality is to know where the end point is. The end point in early prostate cancer should be the removal of all the cancer cells. I heard of a case where two treatments of phototherapy were given through a plastic urinary catheter in an attempt to treat prostate cancer, which was considered sufficient to treat it. The doctor of the patient investigated this patient only two months later for an increasing PSA level, and a referral was made for a prostate biopsy. This showed that the cancer was still there. Needless to say that in this case phototherapy was abandoned and conventional prostate surgery was done.

My conclusion from this is that the dosage of the intravenous photosensitizer, the length of the low-dose treatment exposure and the total number of applications to be given have to be worked out before this method, that may otherwise sound promising, can be recommended. As this one case shows, it is not working reliably at the present time. I consider this still an experimental treatment modality, too risky to use in the treatment of prostate cancer. Finally, when all of this has been worked out, we need a 10-year follow-up trial to prove superior survival data.

Reference regarding phototherapy:
http://www.cancer.org/treatment/treatmentsandsideeffects/treatmenttypes/photodynamic-therapy

High-intensity focused ultrasound (HIFU) Treatment For Prostate Cancer

High-intensity focused ultrasound treatment, also known as HIFU is a treatment that prostate cancer patients are seeking out. The treatment technique is minimally invasive, has low risks of impotence and urinary incontinence and can be done on an outpatient basis. It is a two to three hour procedure that can be done with some mild sedation and spinal anesthesia, and generally men can resume their normal lives immediately after surgery with the knowledge of being cancer-free. Dr. Ian Brown, the medical president of the Niagara HIFU clinic in Niagara Falls, Ontario likens the technique to the effect of a magnifying glass that focuses sunrays on a leaf and burns it. Except there is no sunlight, but a pulse of high-energy ultrasonic waves focused onto a specific area of the prostate.

Temperatures reach approximately 90°C (= 194°F), until the cancer cells are dead. The transducer is equipped with ultrasonic imaging, so the treating physician can see the entire prostate gland on a monitor, and as a result surrounding nerve structures that are responsible for erectile function are not damaged. There is some inconvenience for the patient after the surgery. He has to wear a catheter for two to three weeks until he can urinate on his own. Like any prostate cancer treatment, HIFU also has potential side effects like retrograde ejaculation or urethral fistula development.

Reports state that these side effects are minimalized with HIFU, but they are not eliminated. This treatment is not suitable for every patient. Patients with early stage prostate cancers are suitable candidates. HIFU is not available in the US at present, but has been approved by Health Canada in 2004 based on European data. It is not covered by health insurance, and at $20,000 this new costly option is not affordable for everybody.

The FDA was asked for approval in the US. But according to the FDA panel there is not enough solid data to confirm effectiveness or safety of high-intensity focused ultrasound (HIFU) treatment for prostate cancer. As a result it was not FDA approved in 2014. It is interesting that a high tech solution to prostate cancer has failed at this stage.

Despite the negative assessment by the FDA there are 5-year and 10-year follow-up studies available.

https://www.ncbi.nlm.nih.gov/pmc/articles/PMC4494637/

In this review a 2013 study was cited where the PSA negative survival at 5 years was 81% and at 10 years it was 61%. These data are disappointing and suggest that you are much better off with any other treatment modality except brachytherapy.

Conclusion

Laser therapy has been very useful in other medical applications like removal of skin blemishes, cosmetic surgery (photo rejuvenation), and removal of varicose veins. Laser surgery is also used for refractive eye corneal surgery (LASIK).

Various surgeons like gynecologists and abdominal surgeons use laser surgery because there is less bleeding.

But using laser surgery for cancer treatment is not yet at its prime time, particularly not for prostate cancer. The question is how to define the end point of treating the cancer. How many laser treatments will it take to eradicate the tumor, two, three, four or more? Will it destroy the prostate cancer stem cells, in which case cancer recurrence rates will be low?

In my research of this topic I did not get satisfactory answers to all of my questions. I could not get 5- or 10-year survival rates for MRI guided laser therapy and yet many facilities advertise this as the latest therapy. I consider it still experimental.

I think that any form of laser therapy at this point is not ready for prime time. The same is true for high-intensity focused ultrasound (HIFU) treatment for prostate cancer, despite the approval in Canada I would strongly urge you not to fall into this trap. Be careful about new technologies that have not been tested long enough. As mentioned about

HIFU the 5-year and 10-year survival rates are lower than with any other method, so it clearly is an inferior treatment method.

10-year-survival studies of laser therapy have not been done at this point. Any new treatment modality for prostate cancer has to be proven to be superior in survival figures over a 10-year period.

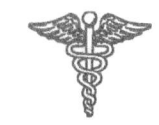

Chapter 14

A Woman's View on Prostate Cancer

Nobody is untouched by the topic "cancer". As women we are seeing fervent support for breast cancer sufferers. There are runs for the cure and the promise of hope that cancer can be beaten. Pink bow emblems convey support for breast cancer patients, victims and their families, but it has been remarkably quiet in women's circles about the male side. Somehow the topic of prostate cancer is not a topic of discussion among women. Not much is heard about support groups, runs for the cure, promises of hope or a ribbon campaign to express support.

It seems that prostate cancer is a topic that is reserved for males. But it is also well known that guys don't really talk about illness. Statistics have it that it is females who are the ones who are seeking medical attention, if they experience health problems. Men by and large have been much more reluctant to make a doctor's appointment and go at great length to postpone physicals, lab tests and procedures. It is not uncommon that women call at the doctor's office and make an appointment for their partners. When they know that something is not right, they are usually the ones insisting that something needs to be done.

With more public information the scenario is slowly changing. Articles about prostate cancer and the need for prostate cancer screening are emerging in male magazines. There are actors and public figures that openly reveal in magazine articles and on the media that they have been diagnosed with prostate cancer.

For men it is a big deal to open up publicly about personal illness, but it is this changing attitude, which promotes more information and educates the male population. Hearing that the fifty-year-old actor Ben Stiller has been diagnosed with prostate cancer in June 2014 is something that men will not simply ignore.

http://people.com/movies/ben-stiller-prostate-cancer-diagnosis-howard-stern-show/

The first reaction will likely be one of shocked surprise: "Wow! Prostate cancer at age 48! And I thought that only old guys get that!" Next the nagging question will come up: "What about me? Could this happen to me too?" When Ben Stiller reveals that he had successful surgery and that his sex life is good again after the surgery, those men who associate prostate cancer surgery with a demise of their sex life will listen up. A condition that they would have rather swept under the rug in past years is all of a sudden not a source of anxiety and the resulting denial. The frankness and honesty of Ben Stiller has very likely done a service to some of those men who sit on the fence, when it comes to prostate cancer screening.

Interestingly enough it will very likely be the female readers who will spot the above-mentioned article in "People's Magazine", but they will also be the ones who will mention it to their male partners and point out the necessity for cancer screening. They are also the ones who have been used to the annual Pap tests and breast exams by mammogram or ultrasound. If women can do it, the men in their lives should hopefully be able to follow suit and have the health screening that applies to males in the form of rectal exams and PSA tests! The only way to assist with an early diagnosis and treatment is information and education. It is important to keep things simple. Men don't read medical textbooks, unless they are health professionals! For this reason alone the most effective vehicle to reach men is information through the media, stressing the need for regular screening.

Despite all better efforts some women will still face the frustration of having a partner who is hard of hearing, when it comes to doctor's visits and exams as well as PSA tests at the lab. As painful as it is, there are limits to what we can do as women: we cannot "snoopervise" our partners. It is tough, but it is a fact! This does not mean that it is now warranted to take the finger-pointing approach of "I told you so", if a male comes down with prostate cancer. Anybody who develops a serious illness like prostate cancer has become utterly vulnerable and needs compassion and unfailing support and not a lecture about failed prevention!

Let's look at a different scenario now. So, your partner is compliant about prostate cancer screening. He is also health conscious and even scrupulous about life style issues. There are no warning signs, not a cloud in the sky, he could be running a commercial for health and fitness and looks younger than his stated age. You should not have any reason to be concerned about his health. Right?

Wrong! Despite all screening and healthy living even the healthiest aging males are not immune to prostate cancer. The older a male is, the more likely he is going to develop prostate cancer. Some are luckier than others, but there are a few males who can develop prostate cancer even before they reach the age of fifty! We have a higher life expectancy now than our ancestors, and cancer has become the illness of the aging. There are warning signs: a rise in the PSA, even if it seems insignificant, is a red flag.

I witnessed exactly that: my husband received lab results, and the PSA had risen a bit, but it was just a small aberration. Six months later it was again slightly higher. This was of concern! But tests are not always consistent: one year later the PSA was slightly lower again. It is an utterly uncomfortable feeling, when test results fluctuate. What should one do? It would be a false sense of security to dismiss this as fluctuations and "minor changes". My husband did not trust the peace either. He decided to take the Oncoblot test, a blood test that screens for twenty-five different kinds of cancer. He wanted to be sure! This test is not inexpensive, but we both agreed that it was a necessary expense to shed some clarity on questions about the rise in the PSA test.

It is needless to say that we did not like to see the results, but they were there: the test pointed to the possibility of prostate cancer, which could affect him within a few years. As shocking as this result was to me, as much I was grateful that my husband had this test. It galvanized him into action and, as we found out soon, it contributed to an early diagnosis. And it cannot be stressed enough, how important an early diagnosis is with prostate cancer!

With this knowledge the next step was an MRI of the prostate. It was not entirely conclusive, as the result pointed to enlargement (hypertrophy) of the prostate.

But there was this small side remark about a "suspicious area", and this was enough to confirm that more investigations were necessary.

The tests were in, and this was a good preparation for a consultation with an urologist. Ray was determined to cover all the bases. His first conversation with a urologist colleague yielded a few more pieces of information. He needed a prostate biopsy first. After that he could be referred for laser ablation. But the laser ablation was just one possibility of treatment.

Getting information about what is the best option is like going shopping for a product. It sounds mundane, but it is not any different: you want what is best for you in your quest for health! The search was only starting, and medical papers are full of information about all sorts of cancer treatments, from the conventional to the wildly unconventional. It is a jungle out there! Some of the articles are anecdotal reports by a few patients, but they are devoid of any type of research. I was interested to know about long-term studies, and not merely a few stories by half a dozen individuals, where a scientific foundation was absent.

For this reason it is best to dig into the websites of universities. One publication was an interesting article about cryotherapy of cancer.

It was approved by the FDA and was described as a very effective form of treatment. It was worth to dig a little deeper, and Ray found a publication about prostate mapping biopsies and subsequent cryoablation therapy. I remember that I read voraciously about prostate cancer therapies on the Internet. After hours of reading, I felt cross-eyed and head tired. But I was also feeling more reassured and less confused. Unless there was a more promising therapy, this procedure would be the most successful one for prostate cancer. It was clear from the statistics that the long-term survival rate was superior and the recurrence rate was much less than with other therapies!

Ray had to wait for a few months to get an appointment at a prominent prostate center in Canada to be seen by one of the urologists there. It was a five-hour drive from our hometown, but it was important for him to have this consultation. He wanted to not miss any important input and did not want to leave any stone unturned. I went with big expectations, as this was a top-notch university affiliated center after all, and Ray was equally confident. It turned out that we were in for nothing impressive. The first question of the receptionist was, whether the patient would be interested to enter into a prospective study. He declined, and I had the feeling that my husband was on the way of being turned into a number in statistics.

Next the doctor saw him. Ray explained his condition to the urologist. He had taken along the elevated PSA results and he also brought the results of the MRI scan, voicing his concern about the suspicious area in the enlarged prostate. The specialist was not too concerned. He wanted to do a rectal examination next first, and after a short exploration he mentioned that he could not even say that the prostate was enlarged! He was not even too sure about a biopsy. Sure, that could be done, but there were a few risks like infection that could land the patient in the emergency. He went so far to declare that in his opinion Ray would not even have a diagnosis of prostate cancer. This could only be confirmed by a biopsy. Ray expressed his interest about a perineal biopsy, and the answer was that this "was not done". They would do a rectal biopsy and "numb him up a bit down there". (Ugh! This did not sound like a nice perspective to me!)

During the conversation my husband attempted to discuss the treatment options, including a mapping biopsy and cryoablation. He had also brought along a copy about this particular publication for the specialist. This was met with a dismissive smile. The specialist stated that it would just be a financial gold mine for the doctor, and he labeled it as a waste of money. It was interesting that he also questioned the scientific validity and statistical relevance of the treatment. With this attitude he probably tossed the paper in the garbage later. He did not sound like he was even informed about the topic at all, was not interested to discuss it, but he parroted what had been pontificated as the "gold standard" of treatment for prostate cancer. In leaving he mentioned that Ray could come back for a biopsy, and here was a prescription for antibiotics before the procedure. This was it; after ten minutes the audience was over. It was obvious that listening was not his strength.

When we walked out of the center, I did not feel confident at all. It was an atmosphere of closed-minded monologue that did not instill trust in me. My husband did not feel any better about this visit either. This was not the place to seek treatment. Family members were appalled and called the visit a waste of time on a beautiful summer day: ten hours on the highway for ten minutes of a consultation. Yes, maybe they were right; however for my husband as well as for me it was important to listen to another medical opinion. Even a disappointment can be positive. At least it points you into the direction you should take on your journey of treating illness in order to get your health back. For Ray it was the decision to choose mapping biopsy and cryoablation therapy.

There are more hurdles on the way. With the knowledge that there is cancer, the clock is ticking. At times I felt an undercurrent of anxiety: how long is it safe to wait till a procedure is done? How fast is the cancer progressing? For my husband the answer was very clear. You don't mess around with cancer! It has to be established at what stage it is. The pathologist always has the last word, whether it comes to assessing cancer in a laboratory setting or seeing the final result, when a person died. In this case the pathologist assesses the type of cancer after a biopsy is taken.

The next logical consequence is the importance to book an appointment with the specialist and go through the necessary steps for this. Since this was a procedure that was not available in our area and not even in our country, it is up to the patient to make all the arrangements and phone calls. Ray is fortunate to have an extremely helpful family physician, and he and his office staff made every effort to provide the out of country specialist with all relevant lab test results. It was a source of comfort and support to get all this help. It was also very reassuring that the office of the specialist was helpful in every possible way, and the specialist also talked to his patient to help clarify any questions.

Nevertheless it still remained a hurdle race to get it all done, as the hospital needs all the records in time. Otherwise the procedure cannot be done!

It is obvious that the partner of the patient is bombarded by a multitude of feelings. After the consultation in Fort Lauderdale, Florida with the specialist I mostly felt relief. My husband was in the hands of a competent and caring physician. He had taken time to discuss details, and one day later he was going to a surgical center for the biopsy. He was asleep. I was awake, and yes, of course it is not easy to wait for a few hours. I would lie, if I would not admit that at times I still worried. I trusted the surgical team, but I also know that surgery and general anesthesia have risks. Our immediate family knew about Ray's condition and the surgery. There were texts from them wishing him well and thinking of us. Still, it is a relief, when your partner is out of surgery, and you hear that everything went very well. The first step is done. After several days the pathology results were available. My husband had early prostate cancer. Contrary to the findings on the MRI scan there were three foci in the prostate. The MRI had only showed one affected area! We had already seen that, when the physician did a high sensitivity ultrasound one day before the biopsy.

It was a surprise, but at least now the results were out. Cryoablation would be the next step a few weeks later.

When your partner becomes a patient, patience is the most important thing for everybody involved. There is no room for doubt or worry. It rather becomes a step-by-step approach of helping with the process of recovery. There are some hurdles like postoperative pain. In Ray's case it was mild pain, and he did not need the prescription of pain medication that the doctor had given him. He did not get any infection, but he needed to drain his bladder by self-catheterization. We did not let this bother us too much in our everyday comings and goings: Ray simply filled a sealed plastic bag with the sterile catheter, lubricant and antibacterial gel. I sunk it into my purse, and we were on our way.

Surgery by cryoablation is a much longer procedure than the mapping biopsy. This meant that I waited several hours, hoping for a successful surgery. I knew that this surgery was much less invasive than a total radical prostatectomy, as there is no incision. Nevertheless there are feelings of uncertainty attached to waiting. After more than three hours it was a relief to see the surgeon come to the waiting area and telling me that my husband was doing well and that the surgery was successful. To the uninitiated who has never seen a patient in recovery right after surgery the first impression can be scary. The patient is still hooked up to a set of beeping monitors, and he is pale, dopey and may be incoherent. He may even feel sick to his stomach. I had worked as a nurse's aide in my university years, and I was prepared for that. All the same this feels different: on this gurney you are not seeing an anonymous patient but your partner. Yes, you need your nerves! This is "only" a day surgery, but now it is up to you to take a post-operative patient home. (For us "home" was a hotel room in Fort Lauderdale close to the hospital).

It is not important that you have nursing skills to look after your partner. Your presence however is important. He will be too tired to say much and will sleep some more, but your silent support of being there for him is the most important part right after surgery. Your partner will not want food, but it is important that you offer him fluids: water and juice may be the best idea. You are also the one who can watch, should there be too much pain or other alarming signs like a fever or bleeding. This is not about nursing, but simply about common sense. You may be in for a disrupted and uncomfortable night, as your partner will experience discomfort due to an indwelling catheter, however the psychological relief that the surgery is done will be making up for this. If he has pain, it can be controlled with a prescription medication. You can also be confident that the next day will be a lot better. Ray was up and about the next morning, he went out for lunch with his doctor, and they discussed the surgery. An afternoon nap is beneficial, but there is no more bed rest necessary, and one day later the patient is able to return home, even if this involves longer travel. This applied to us, as we took a flight in the afternoon back to our hometown in Canada, where we arrived at midnight.

I'm not suggesting, that this is all. Healing is not done in three days! This is a process that takes time. Ray's doctor mentioned that recovery would take approximately six weeks, and Ray found that this projection was correct. The customary workout at the gym was not an option for about two weeks. It caused discomfort. Going for daily walks was enjoyable again after about ten days. It will take a while for your partner to get his bladder control back. Ray did not need the indwelling catheter after day two, but disposable sterile catheters became a standard item for almost four weeks. When they were no longer needed it was a reason to celebrate another milestone of recovery!

After a few weeks, when your partner feels better and has no more discomfort, sex will be on his mind (and probably on your mind as well). When the doctor talked about "sexual rehabilitation" and that the patient needed some "help" in this department, he was not joking! To your partner's utter frustration erections can be initially weak. Even with the fact that cryoablation is sparing the nerve bundles in the prostate, which are responsible for erections, your partner will receive a prescription for those famous "blue pills", Viagra. He will very likely receive the prescription for Cialis as well. For several months these medications will be needed to achieve full erections. For you as well as for him it will be enjoyable to feel intimacy once again without making sex an exercise in frustration. It is important that you take time for each other, and it is yet another step in the process of healing.

You will continue on the journey to health and well-being. He is still a patient, and you also will need patience. Celebrate every small step of progress together, and don't get intimidated by lack of progress or small setbacks.

We experienced that, as my husband developed a urinary tract infection in week five following the surgery. His specialist stated, that it could happen that he hit a "bump on the road". This was no reason to panic, but it meant a prescription for antibiotics and a urine culture later. After one week the road was clear again, and the urine culture was clear as well!

After a surgery for prostate cancer close follow up is necessary in order to stay out of trouble. Your partner will need regular PSA tests every three months. You can help by putting a reminder on his calendar! If there are higher levels, it is not a reason to panic. Take action and consult with the specialist, who will determine whether another biopsy may be needed or not. Not every PSA elevation signals cancer, as the values also can increase with prostatitis.

For all these issues it is important to stay in dialogue with the specialist. You will also talk with your partner, as you are in this together. Together as a team, doctor, patient and the partner of the patient, you can unmask prostate cancer and deal with it!

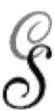

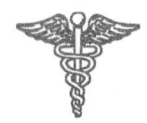

Chapter 15

Ablation Cryotherapy after Mapping Biopsy

Before I review ablation cryotherapy, which is a focal therapy for prostate cancer, I like to review the rational of focal prostate cancer therapy versus more radical procedures like radical prostatectomy or radiotherapy.

The textbook "Campbell-Walsh Urology, Eleventh Edition © 2016 by Elsevier" points out that there is a place for focal prostate cancer therapy, which is placed between the extremes of radical prostate therapy (surgery or radiotherapy) and active surveillance.

This textbook mentions further that not all forms of focal prostate cancer therapies are ready for prime time, based on hundreds of references. The problem with many methods is that they are not more effective than radical prostatectomy in removing prostate cancer or the treatment modality has not been around long enough to prove itself over at least 10 years of follow-up in a larger group of prostate cancer patients.

Here is a brief rundown of these focal therapies.

1. Focal cryoablation: This is the topic of this chapter. But Campbell-Walsh Urology points out that the method is effective in killing prostate cancer provided that the biopsy procedure has been accurate. I will explain below that Dr. Onik from Ft. Lauderdale has introduced the mapping biopsy, which makes the cryotherapy procedure very tumor specific as the whole prostate gland was mapped for cancer. The textbook points out there can be cancer in two or three different places and this would become a problem, if the biopsy would miss one lesion. More about that below.

2. Radiofrequency interstitial tumor ablation: Another method of killing prostate cancer is by the use of radiofrequency interstitial tumor ablation (RITA). With this method a needle-like applicator is introduced through the skin behind the scrotum (perineum) under a local anesthetic. Radiofrequency energy is then delivered under transrectal ultrasound (TRUS) guidance. The transmitted energy heats the tissue around the applicator. When the temperature exceeds 38 degrees Celsius cancer tissue is killed. This method has been investigated as a treatment on its own, by combining this procedure with radiotherapy and as a salvage procedure after radiotherapy failure. The textbook points out that there is not enough long-term experience to recommend this method yet.

3. Focal High-Intensity Focused Ultrasound Ablation: Focal high-intensity focused ultrasound ablation (HIFU) is another method of heating the prostatic tissue for the purpose of killing cancer cells. High intensity ultrasound waves work in the same way as rays of sunlight that pass through a magnifying glass. They are concentrated at a single point, causing a significant temperature rise

around the focal point. The success of this method hinges on the precise localization of the prostate cancer by MRI and biopsy. In one trial 39 men with prostate cancer were treated. After 6 months only 30 were free of their cancer, 4 had to be re-treated, the others were put on active surveillance. There were also complications: 17% had urinary tract infections, 39% had blood in their urine (hematuria), 22% had painful urination (dysuria), 1 had a devastating fistula and 1 was unable to pass urine. The textbook reviewer criticized that the study was ended at 6 months. A long-term follow up would have been required to assess the benefits of this treatment modality. But the conclusion was that "these results are substantially worse than those of radical prostatectomy or radiotherapy".

4. Focal Laser Ablation: This treatment modality is a laser-induced thermal therapy. The technology has been well developed. Laser fibers are introduced into the prostate through needles that puncture the skin behind the scrotum (perineal approach). Nowadays 980-nm diode lasers are increasingly used that reliably destroy cancer cells in the prostate gland. MRI scanning is used during the laser procedure. A feasibility and safety study of this technique has been completed in 2013. The reviewer of the above mentioned textbook (Campbell-Walsh Urology) stated that 33% of the patients had significant erectile dysfunction problems at 6 months following the procedure. There are no 10-year follow-up studies yet, so this method cannot be recommended at this time. The reviewer felt that focal laser ablation would likely become a potential tool for focal therapy of low-risk prostate cancer patients.

5. Photodynamic therapy: Photodynamic therapy (PDT) is a cancer treatment where a low-intensity laser beam activates a previously absorbed photosensitizer

in the prostate cancer to kill the cancer cells. The photosensitizer is given intravenously and within a short time it accumulates in the prostate gland, particularly in the cancer cells. Normal cells can eliminate the photosensitizer rapidly while the cancer cells retain it for a few hours. The laser fibers are introduced through needles that puncture the skin behind the scrotum (perineum) and brought to the prostate cancer under transrectal ultrasonography guidance. The laser frequency is matched to the absorption spectrometer reading of the photosensitizer. This ensures the maximal effect for killing cancer cells. Despite all of the technological development of this method, there are no long-term prostate cancer studies available. The reviewer of the above mentioned textbook summed it up this way: "Oncologic treatment outcomes and side effects have not been well documented because of the limited published studies." As I stated earlier, 10-year follow-up survival data are not available about this method.

Reference: Campbell-Walsh Urology, Eleventh Edition, Copyright © 2016 by Elsevier).

Back to ablation cryotherapy

I came across an article in the 2016 June issue of the health magazine Life Extension regarding a 10-year follow-up of 70 prostate cancer patients who were treated with ablation cryotherapy by Dr. Gary Onik in Ft. Lauderdale, FL.

http://www.lifeextension.com/Magazine/2016/6/Major-Advance-in-Screening-and-Treating-Prostate-Cancer/Page-01

As I indicated briefly in the introduction there was a 100% survival of the prostate cancer patients treated with cryotherapy. 94% were completely free from any recurring prostate cancer. 6% had recurring disease. These kinds of statistics are unheard of with other treatment modalities. The patients' ages were between 45 and 77 years at the time of surgery.

Compare this to a study where prostate cancer was treated with radiotherapy. After 10 years the biochemical disease free survival for low risk patients was 78%, for medium risk 78% and for high risk 62%. This translates into cancer recurrences of between 22% and 38% depending on the risk stratification.

The so-called golden standard procedure (robotic prostatectomy) showed the following: in a study that went on for 5 years there was a 28% overall recurrence rate. When the margins of the prostatectomy were examined, the following amounts of cancer had remained: 23% for low risk patients, 29% for medium risks and 42% for high risks.

When prostate cancer becomes personal

I was attending the 23rd Annual World Congress on Anti-Aging Medicine in Las Vegas (Dec. 11-13) in 2015 where Dr. Mark Rosenberg spoke about the universal cancer marker ENOX-2 that is expressed during embryogenesis (the development of the fetus) and in adulthood only again when cancer develops. A test has been developed to check for the ENOX-2 gene, which becomes positive 5 to 7 years before cancer can be detected clinically. This is called Oncoblot test. Sensitivity of ENOX-2 is high, and false positives are negligible, which makes the ENOX-2 marker ideal for cancer screening. After my return home I decided to contact the company and order the test for myself. I could not believe the result: I was positive for prostate cancer, and yet, I was without any symptoms! I started taking the combination of green tea and capsicum, in case it would be effective in turning the cancer gene off.

I asked my physician for an MRI scan to depict the cancer. This showed one focus in the left lobe of my prostate. There are two lobes, a left and a right one. My PSA values had been in the 1.5 ng/ml range for several years until about 1.5 years ago when the level rose to about 3.0 ng/ml. The Oncoblot test definitely pointed to prostate cancer, and this is something that has to be taken seriously enough to investigate further. At the end of May 2016 my doctor suggested to repeat the PSA test. To my surprise it came back as 8.6 ng/ml. This was getting too much! I needed a prostate biopsy to see what was going on in my prostate gland. At this point I had a positive Oncoblot test for prostate cancer, a lesion confirmed by MRI scan in the left lobe of my prostate and a rising PSA level. I was lucky that I had just read Dr. Onik's 10-year follow-up study following ablation cryotherapy.

I was also coming across a citation from Dr. Allan Stam, a retired Harvard professor who said this about Dr. Gary Onik:

"Dr. Onik is the most innovative cancer specialist in the country." Dr. Stam is a retired professor from Harvard and Tufts Universities and emergency medicine physician who mentored Dr. Onik when he was in college. He is also one of the first patients on which Dr. Onik used cryosurgery (freezing) for prostate cancer. "Cryosurgery is the gold standard for prostate treatment," said Dr. Stam. "Gary always pushes the envelope. He refuses to take other people's opinion that someone cannot be treated. He finds a way. His approach is, 'What are we going to do about it?'"

(Citation from http://www.garyonik.com/doctor-hope).

Contact with Dr. Onik about treating me for prostate cancer

I sent Dr. Onik an email summarizing what I just told you. He suggested that I should give him a call. When we discussed the matter on the phone, he explained to me that I needed to come and see him for a mapping biopsy. This was the only way to know for sure how much cancer was in my prostate and where it was hiding.

Dr. Onik's secretary sent me background material along with questionnaires about my personal health history that I needed to fill out and return. My own physician arranged for me to get blood work and an EKG (heart tracing) in preparation for a general anesthetic. Finally I booked a flight to Fort Lauderdale, and Dr. Onik saw me one day later for an initial assessment, which happened to be on a Sunday. This was news for me, as usually a doctor does not see you on a Sunday in consultation, unless it is an emergency! Dr. Onik went over the history again and proceeded to insert a high sensitivity ultrasound probe into my rectum. His computer screen immediately depicted three lesions, the MRI depicted lesion in my left prostate lobe and two lesions in the right prostate lobe. Dr. Onik was not surprised. He said that this happens a lot that there is more cancer found than initially expected. He also added that prostate cancer is a multifocal disease that often grows in various places at the same time. He further explained that this is why a mapping biopsy is so important, where the total prostate gland is screened for cancer.

Prostate mapping biopsy

When you hear of a biopsy you think that a few needles are inserted into the prostate, and you go home after. This may be the case with a rectal biopsy where only between 16 and 20 needles are used under a local anesthetic.

However, with a mapping biopsy the purpose of the procedure is to do a biopsy every 5 mm (0.2 inches) throughout the entire prostate gland. Some men have an enlarged prostate gland, and much higher numbers of biopsy needles are required to complete the whole grid of biopsies. I had a prostate gland volume of 70 ml as the MRI scan showed, which is more than twice the normal size. Dr. Onik needed 96 biopsies to cover the whole gland. He said that normally only up to 60 biopsies are needed.

With such a high number of needles it is not surprising that this prostate mapping procedure is done in a Medical Center and under a general anesthetic.

I recovered well from this without too much pain. Dr. Onik was surprised that I could not pass urine when I was in the recovery room. So he taught me how to self-catheterize, as he did not want to leave an indwelling catheter in my bladder. I had no problems catheterizing myself several times per day for the next 8 days. Day eight was a big day for me: I could urinate again! After 8 days of not being able to urinate on your own this is a big deal! As all of the organs like rectum, bladder and prostate are closely located together it does not come as a surprise that I had a feeling of pain every time I had a bowel movement or if I urinated.

Even an erection brought on prostate pain, so I knew I was out of commission for having sex with my wife for some time. Finally sex was possible and tolerable two weeks after the mapping biopsy. Little did I know what was to come after the ablation cryotherapy that was much more invasive. Yes, being a patient means that you need patience!

It took a few days before the results of the mapping biopsy came back. The three lesions in my prostate, seen on ultrasound were now confirmed histologically to be prostate cancer. The proof was obvious: 18 (out of the 96) biopsies were positive with grade 6 and grade 7 Gleason score cancer. The rest of the prostate gland was OK. The stage of my prostate cancer was determined to be stage 1c. Dr. Onik said that he could easily treat this. Now I also knew that in my case the combination of green tea and capsicum supplements had not worked. The Internet is full of these home remedies for prostate cancer, but at least in my case I have proof that it did not work.

Ablation cryotherapy and IRE surgery

Dr. Onik told me that he wanted to use two procedures simultaneously in my case to treat my lesions optimally. His concern was the neurovascular bundles that cross through the outer aspect of each lobe of the prostate to the penis. The ablation cryotherapy could destroy them, if he came too close to them, which would result in sexual problems. On the other hand he needed to treat the prostate cancer until all of the cancer cells were dead. The surface antigens would still be intact and would stimulate my immune system to destroy any remaining prostate tumor cells. Dr. Onik has done extensive research regarding the immune response in prostate cancer patients and he was working on a publication with end-stage cancer patients.

The other procedure that was patented in the past and was FDA approved 4 years ago was the IRE surgery.

IRE surgery

Another technique pioneered by Dr. Onik is the NanoKnife or irreversible electroporation (IRE surgery).

http://wwwcancercenter.com/treatments/nanoknife/?source
=BNGPS01&channel=paid+search&invsrc=Non_Branded_
Paid_Search_Bing_General_Search&utm_device=c&utm_
budget=Corporate&utm_site=BING&utm_campaign=Non+
Brand%3ETreatments&utm_adgroup=Interventional+Radio
logy%3ENanoKnife%3EBMM&utm_term=nanoknife&utm_
matchtype=p&k_clickid=da701edf-bddc-41de-bbd9-
c23f4c5e6322&k_profid=422&k_kwid=3835101

This is another tumor ablation method using high voltage electrical impulses that put nano-sized holes into cancer cells, but not into surrounding healthy tissue.

Dr. Onik has been pioneering this procedure on prostate cancer patients, but he has also shown in liver cancer that these methods can double the survival rates, compared to conventional treatment methods. Cancer cells are killed by this method, and the released surface antigens of cancer cells stimulate the immune system to further the healing. The interesting finding in Dr. Onik's past research regarding the IRE surgery is that the neurovascular bundle is not damaged by the IRE surgery within the prostate. With the two lesions in the right prostate lobe Dr. Onik wanted to use mainly IRE surgery, because they were in closer proximity to the neurovascular bundle.

Another hospital stay for the ablation cryotherapy

Other people were celebrating their 2016 summer holiday. I came to Fort Lauderdale for my surgery on August 17, 2016. There was nothing for me to do: I trusted the doctor, and it was time to hand over total control to the hospital team. Since a general anesthetic was used I had no recollection of what happened to me, but I am sure they worked very hard to help me. I woke up feeling kind of dopey like any patient would feel after a general anesthetic.

Otherwise I could feel where my prostate was located, because there was a moderate amount of pain in that region; but this was better than I had expected! I also noticed that I had an indwelling catheter, which was the only thing that did not feel comfortable. That night I tossed and turned because of the indwelling catheter. You feel that there is a foreign body in your bladder (the inflatable rubber ball that keeps the catheter in place). Dr. Onik met me the day after the surgery over lunch in a restaurant. When he saw that there was no bleeding from the catheter, he suggested that I could do self-catheterization again, until it would no longer be needed. He pulled out his computer and showed me on an ultrasound map of my prostate where he treated with IRE and where he used ablation cryotherapy. He was confident that he got all of the cancer destroyed.

But for the next three months he wanted me to take a number of medications.

1. Dutasteride 0.5mg daily for two weeks, then only Mondays and Thursdays for maintenance. This medicine has a long half-life and helps shrink the prostate gland size in patients who have a large prostate (prostate hypertrophy).
2. Metformin 500 mg twice per day to kill stem cells of prostate cancer.
3. Omeprazole (brand names: Prilosec or Losec) 40 mg twice per day to kill stem cells of prostate cancer.
4. Tadalafil (Cialis) 5 mg daily to reduce prostate hypertrophy. I took this for 4 days and developed excruciating lower back pain. Apparently I am one of the 6% to 8% who develop low back pain as a side effect. The receptors in the prostate and in the muscle are the same, so you know it is working. Empirically I found that I could tolerate 5 mg of Cialis every other day without any back pains, but it was still enough for erections.

5. Sildenafil (Viagra) 100mg daily for sex until 3 to 5 months after the surgery. I stopped Viagra after 3 months, but still take 1 tablet every other day together with 5 mg of Cialis. Viagra also helps to reduce prostate hypertrophy.

For 1 month I had to wait before I would use the number 4 and 5 medications. There was no point to attempt sex when I felt discomfort in my prostate with every bowel movement or every urination, and when erections produce a mild pain. But time went by like a blur; I did not even have a desire for sex because there was no feeling like that at all. Getting the message from my body that what previously had been fun was now a painful experience, it seemed that my sex drive had gone into hibernation in the middle of summer, and it started to concern me. Had I become a neutral? When I took the first pill of Cialis I got an amazing erection that lasted, and I realized that I had missed this type of activity. But shortly after there was the back pain episode, which was counter productive.

After that the old habit of sex every other day came back as before the surgery. Often physicians talk about "sexual rehabilitation" after prostate surgery, and the old adage "use it or lose it". This happens to be correct, as initially both, Cialis 5 mg and Viagra 100 mg, were needed to make erections effective. Without medication erections can be a frustrating experience of being either too weak, or nothing is moving in this department. Dr. Onik has seen that it takes between 3 to 5 months following ablation cryosurgery for patients to regain their potency spontaneously. It is yet another point reminding the impatient patient that healing does take its time. Fortunately, in the intervening time drugs like Cialis and Viagra can help the process of sexual rehabilitation.

Self-catheterizations

I knew that there must have been more tissue damage from the surgery when I compared my need for catheterizations after the surgery with the need for catheterization after the mapping biopsy. There was more blood in the urine as the prostate drained blood into the urethra postsurgically. This time it took 30 days before I could urinate spontaneously. After the mapping biopsy it took only 8 days.

Blood in urine

I thought that after 30 days there should be no more blood in the urine. I had hardly 1 week without blood in the urine, when it suddenly reappeared. First I thought that perhaps some blood that was retained in the prostate would have released itself. But when it looked like a male period, I realized that this could no longer be dismissed as normal. Of course this happened on a weekend, and all the offices and urgent care clinics were closed, and so it became a trip to the emergency room of the local hospital. The physician diagnosed a bladder infection, and I had to take a set of antibiotics for 10 days. After 5 days the blood disappeared and my prostate felt normal again. I finished the full 10 days of antibiotics as prescribed. I was a bit apprehensive whether there would be another infection down the road. My physician ordered another urine for culture 5 days after the antibiotics were used up, just in case. This was negative for any infection. Dr. Onik emailed me that urine infections can happen as long as there is an internal wound in the prostate. The prostate takes 6 weeks to heal after the surgery, and during this time some blood can be mixed into urine.

It was a gradual process to return to normalcy: no more catheters by 4 weeks, no more infection, and 6 weeks had passed. Sex works with the help of pills, but I am waiting for normal, spontaneous sex to return.

Follow-up

Like with any health condition it is important to stay compliant and vigilant. The follow-up consists of monitoring PSA levels every 3 months for 2 years. After two years PSA levels are monitored every 6 months. If there was extensive prostatic cancer removed you may be advised at the end of the first year to have a repeat mapping biopsy. If the PSA level stays low nothing further has to be done, but if at any time the PSA level increases another mapping biopsy is required. Dr. Onik said that a PSA of 3.0 ng/ml or below would be acceptable. The value for cryotherapy is higher than with radical prostatectomy, as much more of the normal prostate tissue is left behind, which produces a certain amount of PSA.

On Nov. 15, 2016 I had two tests. The first was a repeat PSA test, which came back as 0.9 ng/ml (down from 8.6 ng/ml). The second test was a repeat Oncoblot test. This came back as negative for prostate cancer. This was a double reason to celebrate. It meant that the prostate cancer was successfully removed. I had two more PSA tests since then: Dec 30, 2016: PSA 0.92 ng/ml and on March 30, 2017: the PSA was 0.95 ng/ml. I will continue to follow the protocol with 3-monhtly PSA blood tests for 2 years. After the two years, I'll go for PSA testing every six months. With regard to the Oncoblot test, I would be considered cancer free for 7 to 8 years after which it should be tested again. To be on the cautious side, I will have the Oncoblot test in 5 years from my cryoablation surgery.

Conclusion

There are several points that impressed me with ablation cryotherapy.

1. It starts with the mapping biopsy, which gives an exact histological picture of any prostate cancer in your prostate. This provides the roadmap for the surgeon to treat any lesions that are found in the biopsy with ablation cryotherapy. While the biopsies are taken there is transrectal ultrasound guidance (TRUS) using a rectal probe. This helps in locating the cancer 3-dimensionally.
2. Like the mapping biopsy the ablation cryotherapy is done under general anesthetic. The same lesions found with the mapping biopsy are treated now with special Argon sounds, and temperature probes measure the temperature to make sure the cancer was frozen long enough. This is repeated one more time to be certain that all cancer cells are killed.
3. For cancer lesions too close to the neurovascular bundle to be removed with cryotherapy, the surgeon can use the alternative, IRE or also called NanoKnife. It had been researched in dogs and later in humans that it will eradicate cancer cells, but not normal cells. It also does not attack the neurovascular bundle. Between the two procedures the entire cancer within the prostate can be removed safely.
4. This means that the side effects are much less than with conventional prostate surgery. The erectile dysfunction is only temporary for 3 to 5 months, but Cialis and/or Viagra can be titrated to achieve normal sex until your own erections come back. There is no effect on the rectum and no sign of bladder leakage. Problems urinating are

only temporary in the beginning and can be overcome with self-catheterization or with an indwelling catheter for a period of time. The end result is that the patient is back to normal, and the prostate cancer is removed.

When I compared all of the other prostate cancer procedures to ablation cryotherapy, I came to the conclusion that ablation cryotherapy was the best solution for me. It is straightforward, cancer specific and works with the least amount of damage to the normal surrounding tissue. The 10-year survival was 100% with a tumor free rate of 94%. Another advantage of this method is that anytime the PSA would be elevated in the follow-up blood tests, the mapping biopsy could be repeated and if a recurrent cancer should be found, the ablation cryotherapy could be done again.

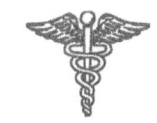

Chapter 16:

Chemotherapy of Prostate Cancer

Chemotherapy for prostate cancer is considered when there is evidence of metastases that do not respond to radiotherapy. Chemicals with strange names like docetaxel, mitoxantrone, paclitaxel, epirubicin, estramustine and cabazitaxel are used to stop cancer cells from dividing. You can read more about them here:

http://www.cancerresearchuk.org/about-cancer/prostate-cancer/advanced-cancer/advanced-treatment/chemotherapy/chemotherapy-drugs

The concept of chemotherapy is a double-sided sword, as the immune cells will also stop dividing, the hair follicles stop producing hair and the gut lining cells stop multiplying when chemotherapy is given. The end results are the familiar side effects of chemotherapy: vomiting, diarrhea, fever from infections and hair loss. There is no objective evidence of prolongation of life except for a few months here and there. But this is offset by premature deaths from septicemia as a result of the suppression of the immune system. Chemotherapy also does not improve the quality of life and does not lead to permanent cures. The chemotherapeutic agents are insanely expensive, and it has become big business to produce them. From a theoretical viewpoint it also does not make sense. Chemotherapeutic agents are releasing free radicals, which do damage to the cancer cells. As we will hear in the next chapter, they do not touch the cancer stem cells. But they leave the body weakened from the free radical damage. The question is whether the body that is already weakened from the cancer is in a position to rebuild itself after the waves of chemotherapy treatments have gone through it. At the end the chemotherapy-resistant cancer stem cells simply multiply and the cancer comes back with a vengeance.

Drug companies are supporting oncologists

Chemotherapy drugs are often very toxic and less effective in treating cancer successfully than what the drug companies promise. No private person purchases chemotherapy drugs, and the drug companies depend on oncologists to support their products. One way to do that is to give the oncologists a good deal on the drugs when they buy them wholesale. They can subsequently charge the full retail price to Medicare. This works well in a private office setting. In a hospital setting it helps the hospital to make a profit, but not the oncologist.

Basically, we are talking about various forms of kickbacks. It is almost criminal to use drugs as toxic as chemotherapeutic drugs on patients, if the motivation is nothing else but profit thinking. The use of chemotherapeutic drugs should solely be based on the objective need of the patient.

http://www.cancerdefeated.com/this-secret-hustle-has-cancer-doctors-rolling-in-dough/1124/

Conclusion

Chemotherapy is problematic as the cancer drugs do not only kill cancer cells, but also normal cells and in particular the immune system cells. The end result are hair loss, vomiting from irritating the gut and possible life threatening infections due to the suppression of the immune system. The design of the anti- cancer treatment with chemotherapy is a misfit between the cancer drugs and the so-called therapeutic effect. Chemotherapists simply talk about side effects to downplay the non-specificity of the treatment of chemotherapy. They also do not tell you that chemotherapy has no effect on the cancer stem cells and that chemotherapy resistant prostate cancer cells will be the leftover after chemotherapy is finished. This is what kills the patient at the end.

I was looking for what 10-year survival rates for chemotherapy would be, but I could not find any. Sadly, the longest survivors after chemotherapy live only for about 1 year.

Like with radiation the prostate cancer stem cells are resistant to chemotherapy.

https://www.ncbi.nlm.nih.gov/pmc/articles/PMC4708185/

I conclude that chemotherapy has not much value at all in the treatment of prostate cancer. A patient may be better off without chemotherapy and just palliative medication for pain.

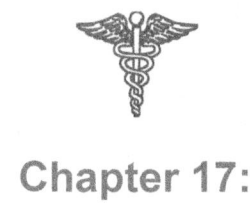

Chapter 17:

Prostate Cancer Stem Cells

If you want to cure cancer, you need to know about cancer stem cells. In my opinion the most important breakthrough in cancer research in the last decade has been the realization that standard cancer treatment protocols don't work very well. They consisted of using surgery, radiotherapy and chemotherapy. Surgery is effective for early cancer. But radiotherapy and chemotherapy have been disappointing. Instead cancer immunotherapy has emerged as the missing link in the last 10 years. The full truth about cancer can only be understood, when we realize that most, if not all solid tumors are having their own cancer stem cells (CSC). In the past this was only recognized for leukemia, largely because of a lack of testing methods for solid tumors. We now have at least two methods of proving the existence of CSCs in solid tumors, as I will explain in more detail below. Using this new cancer stem cell concept, cancer can only be cured when the CSCs are eradicated.

New assays for cancer stem cells

Originally the concept of regular stem cells was proven in mice by radiating them and injecting bone marrow cells into them to rescue them.

http://www.cancerresearchuk.org/about-cancer/prostate-cancer/advanced-cancer/advanced-treatment/chemotherapy/chemotherapy-drugs

When the animals were sacrificed colonies were detected in their spleens that were of the same cell type as the injected stem cells. This new thinking revolutionized the treatment of leukemia. Bone marrow transplants were introduced that allowed in some cases a cure for leukemia. Presently there is a new wave of stem cell treatment applications for a variety of conditions.

With regard to developing an assay for cancer stem cells in solid tumors researchers took a strain of hairless mice that are known to be immune deficient (they lack thymus derived lymphocytes or T cells). They are officially called nude mice.

https://en.wikipedia.org/wiki/Nude_mouse

When human cancer stem cell samples are injected into them, they develop the original cancer of human origin, and the nude mice succumb to metastases.

Histologically the tumors in these mice are the same as the original human cancer. Another mouse model was also shown to be equally effective in demonstrating CSC activity. The immune system of regular laboratory mice can be paralyzed with prior chemotherapy treatment. Using these chemotherapy pre- treated mice the CSC assay works very similar to the one using nude mice.

https://www.ncbi.nlm.nih.gov/pmc/articles/PMC2827660/

If isolated cancer stem cells are injected into the nude mouse or immunosuppressed mouse model, cancer cells, such as prostate cancer stem cells will grow in a short time, which have the same appearance histologically as in prostate cancer biopsies from a man affected by prostate cancer.

Cancer stem cells in prostate cancer

Prostate cancer seems to originate from a cancer stem cell (CSC). The CSC has no androgenic receptors contrary to the majority of prostate cancer cells. This may be the reason why radiotherapy, hormone ablation therapy and chemotherapy do not affect CSCs in prostate cancer. Ultimately this is the reason why the patient dies when the resistant CSCs multiply in the end stage.

One of the important new insights into cancer is that CSCs have the same surface antigen components as the cancer cells despite the difference in other receptors like hormone receptors. One of the techniques of killing prostate cancer is ablation cryotherapy using Argon applicators that freeze the cancer cells, followed by thawing them again.

https://www.cancer.org/cancer/prostate-cancer/treating/cryosurgery.html

The interventional radiologist, Dr. Gary Onik was the inventor of this technique.

http://www.garyonik.com/the-doctor

Using temperature probes this can be controlled and is done at least twice. This will eliminate all prostate cancer including the prostate CSC. At the same time it will stimulate human T cells to recognize the cancer cell surface antigens as foreign and mount an immune reaction to eliminate any remaining cancer cells and all the CSCs. Prior to treating with cryotherapy the cancer cells were secreting substances that disabled the immune cells from recognizing prostate cancer as foreign cells. Now the cryosurgery does a double task: this therapy kills cancer cells and CSC and vaccinates patients against their specific tumors. This eradicates metastases and either cures the cancer or prolongs survival.

http://www.garyonik.com/doctor-hope

Irreversible electroporation and cancer stem cells

Another technique pioneered by Dr. Onik is the Nano-Knife, http://emjreviews.com/wp-content/uploads/Pushing-the-Limits-with-Nanoknife%C2%AE-A-Promising-New-Technology-in-Localised-Prostate-Cancer-Managem.pdf or irreversible electroporation (IRE). This is another tumor ablation method using high voltage electrical impulses that put nano-sized holes into cancer cells, but not into surrounding healthy tissue. Dr. Onik has been pioneering prostate cancer treatment, but he has also shown that IRE treatments of liver cancer can double the survival rate compared to conventional treatment methods. Again, CSC and cancer cells are killed by this method and the released surface antigens of cancer cells stimulate the immune system to further the healing.

Other solid tumors and cancer stem cells

In the last 10 years new methods have been developed to demonstrate the existence of CSCs in many solid tumors. Both the cryotherapy ablation method as well as the IRE method that stimulate the immune system in the sense of a cancer vaccination, https://www.cancer.gov/about-cancer/causes-prevention/vaccines-fact-sheet are not only effective in prostate cancer. It works for most solid tumors such as pancreatic cancer, liver cancer, melanoma, breast cancer, colon cancer and many more.

These new evolving cancer therapies are essentially avoiding the trap of chemotherapy and radiotherapy where only more resistant cancer cells are produced. By removing the original cancer with cryosurgery and/or IRE the immune system is specifically stimulated to recognize the surface antigens of the cancer cells and the CSCs at the same time. With this cancer vaccination process the CSCs are eliminated, and this prevents new cancer cell clones (metastases) from developing. Dr. Onik has recently treated incurable cancer patients and has a cure rate of about 30% (personal communication) in patients who previously would all have died. Others are partial cures, where patients live much longer than anticipated. Using these techniques it is possible in many cases to cure end stage cancer. This has been done with end stage prostate cancer, liver cancer and pancreas cancer, cancers that are extremely difficult to treat otherwise.

https://prostatecancernewstoday.com/2014/12/11/focal-cyroablation-improves-prostate-cancer-survival-and-quality-of-life/

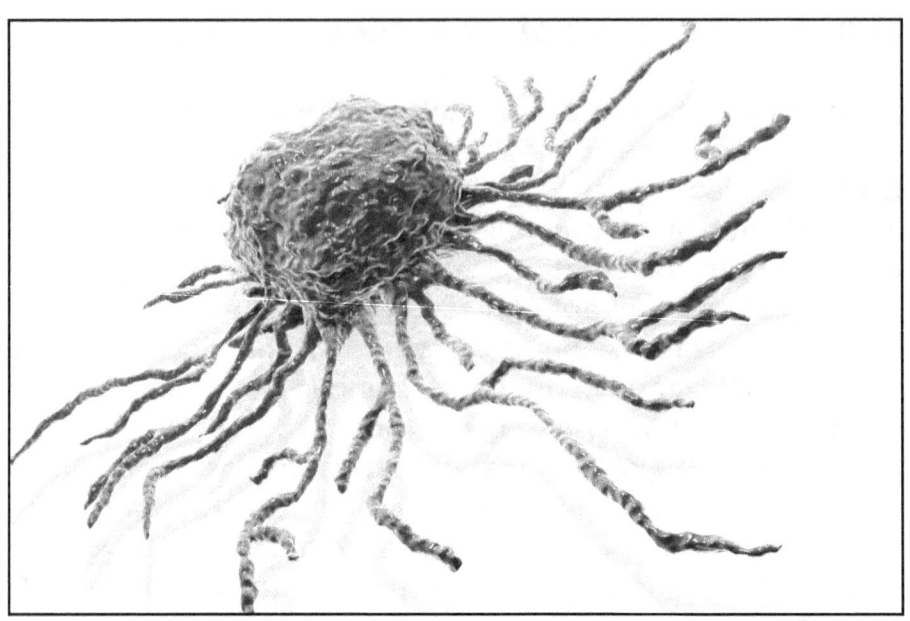

Conclusion

Cancer seems to develop out of cancer stem cells that are abnormal cells with genetic mutations. They are resistant to chemotherapy and radiotherapy, but respond to surgery, to cryotherapy and to irreversible electroporation (IRE). The advantage of cryotherapy and IRE is that the tumor and the cancer stem cells are removed, but at the same time the killed cancer cells stimulate the immune system to produce cancer-fighting antibodies that kill metastases and any remaining cancer stem cells. Although initially shown to be effective in prostate cancer patients, this method has since been tested in terminal cancer patients with pancreatic cancer, melanoma, liver cancer, brain cancer and many more solid tumor types.

Cancer is a disease where the immune system is weak, and it is logical that immunotherapy will be useful in its treatment. Surgery can only be successful, if the entire tumor is removed, which is only possible in stage 1 or stage 2 cancer development. Radiotherapy leaves cancer cells and CSC behind that will become resistant to treatment. Chemotherapy has the dismal prospect of killing the immune system and ultimately the patient. It appears that cryotherapy (and/or IRE) and the associated immunotherapy are the way of future cancer treatments. This is the most important breakthrough in cancer research during the last ten years.

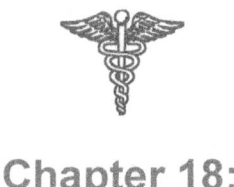

Chapter 18:

Prevention of Prostate Cancer

In this section I like to address the things men can do to prevent prostate cancer. If you are young enough, let's say in your 30's or 40's there is enough time to work on prevention. Keep in mind though that prevention is only effective to a certain degree on a personal level. But on a population level it will definitely make a significant difference.

Here are the preventative factors to keep in mind.

1. Afro American men and prostate cancer

Afro American men normally have twice the risk of getting prostate cancer than white men. But Afro American men were found to have 71% less prostate cancer, if their serum 25-hydroxyvitamin D level was at least 30 ng/ml or higher.

https://www.ncbi.nlm.nih.gov/pubmed/26047130

2. University of Arizona Cancer Center criticizes vitamin D3 studies

A publication from the University of Arizona Cancer Center in Jan. 2016 is more critical of the evidence regarding vitamin D3 and the claim that it lowers cancer rates.

https://www.ncbi.nlm.nih.gov/pubmed/26918035

They reviewed the cancer literature and found that for colorectal cancer there is a clear inverse relationship between serum 25(OH)D levels on the one hand and rates and mortality of colorectal cancer on the other hand. However, with breast cancer the literature was more divided. Only higher vitamin D levels were related to a lower risk for progression of breast cancer and a lower mortality rate.

For prostate cancer conditions were similar with the exception of a study using 4000 IU of vitamin D3 per day, which inhibited progression of prostate cancer. The key is to take a high enough vitamin D3 dose to make it effective not only against prostate cancer, but against other cancers as well. My recommendation is to start taking 5000 IU of vitamin D3 daily. After 3 months ask your doctor to send you for 25-hydroy-vitamin D blood levels. Your goal should be a vitamin D level of 50 to 80 ng/ml.

Adjust your vitamin D3 intake according to the lab results. Vitamin D3 is safe, but better make sure your blood absorbed enough of the supplement you take. There are slow absorbers and fast absorbers.

3. Effects of vitamin D3 on cancer prevention

This Chinese study examined the effects of vitamin D3 on cancer prevention.

https://www.ncbi.nlm.nih.gov/pubmed/23895685

It found that vitamin D3 combines three specific actions in one. Vitamin D3 is anti-proliferative meaning that it stops uncontrolled cell division.
Secondly, it has an apoptotic (cell death) effect, which means it supports the removal of cells that are dying. If they are dying, but not removed, cancer can occur from these cell remnants. The third effect of vitamin D3 is that it has differentiating effects in several malignant cell types. When cancer cells are non-differentiated (=more immature cells) cancer can multiply quickly. When cancer cells are becoming more specific cells uncontrolled multiplication is much more difficult. This is an effect that controls the speed by which cancer cells divide and how quickly cancer metastasizes. Three actions in one from vitamin D3! I took my vitamin D3 today, did you take yours?

4. Avoid getting a beer-belly:

You heard the expression "beer belly". It is an unflattering term for increased abdominal girth, usually referring to males. It is quite often that this picture is found in middle-aged men who consume more beer than what is good for them, but they may also mill around the hot dog stands at the ball game instead of being physically active. Any leftover calories are stored as belly fat, which protrudes their stomach. But a tummy looking like a "male pregnancy" is dangerous! There is a big difference between belly fat and body fat. Belly fat is metabolically much more active. Body fat is more sessile. It is the belly fat that has to go first, as this has been shown to be associated with heart attacks, strokes and diabetes.

http://www.nature.com/nrgastro/journal/v2/n6/full/ncpgasthep0197.html

Originally it was thought that excessive weight would best be measured with the body mass index (BMI). But subsequently it was shown that athletes with well-developed muscles could have BMI's that were in the overweight (between 25.0 and 30.0) or even obese category (more than 30.0). Also, some people with heavy bones can have excessive BMI values despite the fact that things are normal, based on other measurements. The new measurement is the old fashioned abdominal girth to hip ratio.

https://www.hsph.harvard.edu/obesity-prevention-source/obesity-definition/abdominal-obesity/

You measure the abdominal girth, the hip girth and divide the abdominal girth by the hip girth. Normally this should be 80% (=0.8) or less for women and 90% (=0.9) or less for men. But a person with a beer belly will have ratios of 1.2 or 1.5. This is where it shows that there is a problem. If that person has blood tests, there would very likely be findings of elevated triglycerides, lowered HDL cholesterol (the protective cholesterol) and elevated LDL cholesterol (the bad cholesterol). But it does not stop there. We know from studies that often the fasting insulin level is elevated in the sense of hyperinsulinism. In fact that person often has the metabolic syndrome, which is a characteristic change of the metabolism in an obese person. The blood is thicker with clotting factors floating around, there are inflammatory kinins that circulate and all of these factors can cause hardening of the arteries.

Why is a beer belly dangerous?

There are not only cardiovascular risks on the long-term causing heart attacks and strokes down the road. There is a danger of fat deposits in the liver, called fatty liver disease.
In time this can turn into liver cirrhosis and in some cases develops into liver cancer. Because belly fat causes inflammation in the system, including in the lining of the blood vessels, this can in time also affect the immune system, weakening it and eventually allowing cancer to develop. Common cancers that are associated with obesity are breast cancer, ovarian cancer and uterine cancer in women, prostate cancer in men and pancreas and colon cancer in both sexes.

http://www.webmd.com/cancer/news/20080214/
overweight-obesity-linked-to-cancers#1

In men beer bellies produce a lot of estrogen, the female hormone. The reason for this is that fat tissue contains the enzyme aromatase, which metabolizes male hormones into estrogen. Estrogen in men is only good in traces, but when it is massively produced it will counter testosterone and cause heart attacks and strokes.

What can be done about a beer belly?

We need to understand how beer bellies develop. One of the sources of fat from beer bellies is the consumption of foods that contain a lot of sugar and fructose. Food manufacturers have been diligent in mixing high fructose corn syrup into sugary drinks and into a myriad of processed foods.

Sugar itself can only be processed and stored until the glycogen stores in the liver and the muscles are filled. The liver metabolizes a surplus of sugar into triglycerides and LDL cholesterol. This is also the case for any fructose that comes from metabolized sucrose (table sugar) and from the high fructose corn syrup popular with the food processing industry. One problem is that fructose can only be processed by the liver, while glucose gets directly taken up by cells with the help of insulin.

https://www.ncbi.nlm.nih.gov/pubmed/23031075

The surplus of fructose is mostly used to metabolize into triglycerides and LDL cholesterol before it is stored as fat in fat cells. Unfortunately a lot of the fat will end up between the guts, in the liver as fatty liver and in the beer belly, a metabolically more active form of fat.

The sad part is that in the 1960's I have seen the German economic wonder ("Wirtschaftswunder") where many men in the mid-fifties to mid- sixties died as a result of obesity and subsequent heart attacks and strokes. At that time it was thought that Germans, having been starved during World War II, lived it up in the late fifties and 1960's to the point where they ate whatever they could get hold of: cakes, fatty cheeses, rich cakes with whipped cream, fatty foods like pork roasts and beef. They also consumed loads of bread, buns, pasta and sugar. Margarine also became popular with its hydrogenated fatty acids that also contained free radicals. The end result was that they gained weight, did not exercise and developed their beer bellies.

Since the 1980's when low fat/high carbs became popular to replace saturated fatty acids that were supposed to be responsible for heart attacks, strokes and obesity, obesity continued to steadily increase. Sure, the hydrogenated fatty acids did not help and should be cut out. But the bigger problem was the consumption of high fructose corn syrup and over-consumption of high glycemic-index carbohydrates.

Here is the solution of what to do get rid of the beer belly

a) Remove sugar and high fructose corn syrup from your diet.
b) The second effective step is to cut out as many empty starches that you can. Cut out white rice, bread, sweets, cookies, cakes, ice cream and pasta. The reason for this is that these starchy foods get metabolized in the gut into sugar, which causes an insulin response. The extra insulin is responsible for developing inflammation in the arteries, which eventually leads to heart attacks and strokes.
c) Exercise on a regular basis. This will produce HDL cholesterol, the protective cholesterol, which balances LDL cholesterol.
d) Perhaps the most important step is to rebalance your food intake. With this I mean that you replace high glycemic-index carbs with low glycemic-index carbs. This means you will eat a lot of salads, steamed and raw vegetables, and fruit. This gives you a lot of extra fiber, which your system needs to slow down the rate of sugar absorption, helps you to lower LDL cholesterol and helps you to detoxify your body in the gut where toxins are bound to fiber.
e) If you are heavily into alcoholic drinks, this is another source of refined carbohydrates that gets metabolized

into LDL cholesterol and triglycerides. It can also cause fatty liver disease and liver cirrhosis. A moderate consumption of alcohol (one drink for women per day and two drinks for men per day) lowers the risk of heart attacks and strokes, while excessive alcohol intake increases the risk.

http://www.livestrong.com/article/269045-does-alcohol-raise-cholesterol-levels/

f) Bioidentical hormone replacement may be something you have not heard about. But if you are a woman above the age of 40 or a man above the age of 50, chances are that your natural hormone production from the ovaries or adrenal glands (in a woman) or from your testicles or adrenal glands (in a man) are no longer keeping up with the demands of regular life. Part of the aging process is that the production of our sex hormones slows down shortly before menopause in women and shortly before andropause in men. This will not only manifest itself in hot flashes and sleep disturbance in women or in erectile dysfunction and grumpiness in men; it will eventually lead to a lack of energy metabolism in the heart, the brain and other organ systems that have sex hormone receptors. A lack of hormones translates into yet another cause for heart attacks, strokes and certain cancers. This is an area where conventional medicine disagrees with anti-aging medicine. But it is my experience from years in general practice that heart attacks, strokes, colorectal cancer and pancreatic cancer in both sexes, cancer of the breasts, uterus and ovaries in women and prostate cancer in men are indeed more common when natural hormone production has declined. For an aging male it means to see your doctor for a testosterone level. If this is below 350 ng/dL ask for testosterone replacement. Other sources say that testosterone replacement should started below 500 ng/dL and brought to high normal levels of 700 to 800 ng/dL. It will prevent prostate cancer, not cause it.

https://www.sciencedaily.com/releases/2016/05/160507143326.htm

On the other hand, when bioidentical hormone replacement is given, the metabolism of all cells will return to normal and the likelihood of not developing all these illnesses at an earlier time is diminishing as well. It is not a panacea for eternal life, but it will add significant longevity without premature disabilities, which is what we all need.

Summary

Although weight gain around the waistline is common these days and increased mortality due to heart attacks, strokes and cancer is common, we do not have to accept this as the new norm. We need to assess our food intake habits, cut out the items that contribute to the beer belly and ask ourselves what other change in lifestyle we need to make in order to improve our body shape and our energy metabolism. Life is too precious to just throw away years of fruitful living in our golden retirement years. Work on these factors in midlife or even in younger years and you can enjoy disease-free aging.

5. Healthy nutrition will help prevent prostate cancer

In North America we tend to eat too much beef and red meats. This includes sausages, breakfast meats and pork. Here is a website that explains in more detail what a good diet is:

**https://zerocancer.org/learn/current-patients/maintain-qol/
diet-and-nutrition/**

One interesting observation is that the prostate cancer rates among Asian countries are lower than in the west. Similarly Asian immigrants to the US are experiencing higher prostate cancer rates as their diets are changing.

https://www.ncbi.nlm.nih.gov/pmc/articles/PMC3814115/

Another good source of diet would be a Mediterranean diet with lots of vegetables and olive oil. Don't think that you are 100% protected from prostate cancer, if you switch to a Mediterranean diet. There can be genetic factors and the influence of environmental factors like xenoestrogens that are also causing disease. Still, it is important to choose a healthy lifestyle. If you are diagnosed with prostate cancer, a switch in diet from a not-so-good diet to a healthier diet can definitely help. Your body will be in a much better shape to fight any type of illness.

6. Western diet bad for prostate cancer

We just heard that it matters what eating habits you have. Here are two more studies that found that it mattered.

1. A study from the Harvard T.H. Chan School of Public Health followed 926 men aged 40 to 84 who were diagnosed with prostate cancer, but whose cancer had not yet spread. The patients were monitored for approximately 10 years. The diet of the patients was analyzed 5 years after the diagnosis of the prostate cancer using detailed questionnaires. Men who followed a Westernized diet with red meat, refined grains, high-fat dairy products and processed foods had a probability

of dying that was 2.5-times higher than men who were on the healthiest diet. In terms of dying from any cause the men on the Westernized diet had a 1.5- fold higher risk than the men on the healthiest diet.

https://www.hsph.harvard.edu/news/press-releases/
western-diet-may-increase-death-risk-after-prostate-
cancer-diagnosis/

The same recommendations that are made regarding prevention of cardiovascular disease to the general public are the very same dietary recommendations that helped men with diagnosed, but localized prostate cancer to keep the prostate cancer from spreading and killing the patients.

Dr. Jorge Chavarro, the lead investigator said that men who have been diagnosed with prostate cancer should choose a Mediterranean type diet with vegetables and fruit, fiber and less dairy products and less meat. This will help them improve their chances of survival.

Another study published in Cancer Prevention Research (April 14, 2015) found that green tea catechins in capsule form were effective in preventing the development of prostate cancer in 23 of 26 men; at the time of enrolment into the study they all had high-grade prostatic intraepithelial cancer and three men developed prostate cancer after one year of observation. In the control group who only received placebo pills 10 men came down with prostate cancer. The patients on green tea catechins also had a reduction of their PSA (a prostate marker) values in comparison to the placebo group.

2. The question is how the Mediterranean diet can protect men from prostate cancer compared to men consuming a Standard American diet. And the same question can be asked regarding the green tea catechins. At the 23rdAnnual World Congress on Anti-Aging Medicine in

Las Vegas (Dec. 11-13) Dr. Mark Rosenberg may have answered this question. He spoke about the ENOX-2 gene located on the X-chromosome, which is expressed during embryogenesis and then in adulthood only again when cancer develops. A test has been developed to check for the ENOX-2 gene, which becomes positive 5 to 7 years before cancer can be detected clinically. This is called Oncoblot test.

http://www.oncoblotlabs.com/wp-content/
uploads/2014/06/Doctor-Deck-Draft-v11-RD.pdf

As sensitivity of ENOX-2 is high and false positives are negligible, this makes the ENOX-2 marker suitable for cancer screening. There are various isoelectric points for various cancer tissues, so the lab physician can tell the treating physician from which tissue a positive cancer test originates. The interesting thing is that a combination of green tea and capsicum has been able to suppress the expression of the gene in a significant amount of men followed, and the cancer gene was turned off. Corresponding biopsy samples showed that the cancer cells had disappeared. This is an entirely new concept.

Summary: We are entering a new era, where cancer is seen from a different angle. It appears that there are cancer inducing foods and chemicals (called carcinogens) that turn cancer genes like the ENOX-2 gene on. But there are other substances like catechins in green tea and capsicum (derived from hot pepper) that can turn off cancer genes (like the ENOX-2 gene). In this light the effect of green tea in the second trials described above and the effect of the Mediterranean diet regarding the first trial seem to make more sense. It underlines the old principle that prevention is more powerful than any attempt to heal.

7. Fiber lowers prostate cancer risk

French researchers published a study that involved 3313 men and lasted for 12.6 years on average. It involved the consumption of insoluble fiber; specifically, the quantity, source and types of fiber consumed were analyzed. The study started in 1994 and went on until 2007. 139 men developed prostate cancer during that time. The research-ers compared the men who consumed the top 25% fiber with the group of 25% men who consumed the lowest amount of fiber. The surprising result was that the top fiber consuming men had 53% less prostate cancer when compared to the lowest fiber-consuming group.

The men had been analyzed with food questionnaires on at least three occasions during the study period. They were part of a larger nutritional study called SU.VI. MAX (Suppleméntation en Vitamines et Minéraux Anti-oxydants).

In addition the fiber type was analyzed and it was found that insoluble fiber such as the fiber of legumes was most protective in terms of prostate cancer prevention.

What does this mean in practical terms? Meat and potatoes have no fiber. Instead eat a lentil soup, beans, a vegetable chili, a Middle Eastern dish of chickpeas, a pea soup (good in winter), just to give you some suggestions.

8. Prostate cancer recurrence linked to obesity

Here is an interesting study that examined recurrence rates of prostate cancer depending on how overweight or obese the men were.

Prostate cancer affects a significant percentage of male patients in the higher age group. Early diagnosis and treatment has shown good success rates. Early surgery in the form of a radical prostatectomy has given patients virtually a new lease on life. Radiotherapy as an alternative form of treatment has been an option for those who could not undergo surgery. Once the treatment is completed there is reason for optimism, if the tumor could be removed in total.

Dr. Sara Strom, PhD and research colleagues from the M.D. Anderson Cancer Center in Houston, Texas analyzed findings of 873 patients over the course of 14 years with localized prostate cancer who had received external beam radiotherapy as their sole treatment. The objective was to determine, whether all patients were doing well, or whether some were more at risk. It turned out that those who had a normal body weight fared best. 27% of them experienced a recurrence of the disease. Those who were overweight had recurrence rates that jumped to 55%. And those who were obese were most severely affected with recurrence rates of 99%. The researchers believe that there is a difference of tumor behavior between patients with normal body weight and those who are overweight or obese.

The authors felt that future studies will be needed to evaluate the relationship of obesity with dietary factors, genetic modifiers of steroid androgen metabolism, insulin and insulin like growth factors. The authors thought that this would clarify the underlying mechanism of action in the development of prostate cancer.

In the meantime it is clear to me that the same metabolic and hormonal changes that were described under the "beer belly" above are also operative here. In other words, if you are overweight or obese and you want to survive longer you must cut out sugar and starchy foods. I have summarized this in a blog:

http://www.askdrray.com/sugar-as-a-cause-of-cancer/

9. Vitamin D3 prevents prostate cancer and improves survival of it

Although I mentioned vitamin D3 before, I like to add the following studies that further confirm the importance of taking vitamin D3.

A study showed that higher vitamin D3 leads to better prostate cancer survival. https://www.ncbi.nlm.nih.gov/pubmed/26809275 The article appeared in the medical journal Cancer Epidemiology, Biomarkers & Prevention. The Alpha-Tocopherol, Beta-Carotene Cancer Prevention Study was used to zero in on prostate cancer. 1000 subjects in that study had prostate cancer at the time of enrolment. Over the course of the 23-year study just over 360 subjects died from prostate cancer. Serum 25-hydroxyvitamin D levels were obtained at the time of enrolment into the study. The participants of the study also completed food questionnaires. This documented the uptake of vitamin D3 from food.

Results of the study were as follows:

Those whose vitamin D levels were among the top 20% of the group had a much better survival than the bottom 20% of vitamin D levels among the group. The top vitamin D level group survived 28% better than the bottom group!

The authors noted that the finding of their study has important implications. Disease specific mortality, in this case prostate cancer is significantly reduced in the presence of vitamin D3 supplementation. The authors are of the opinion that all prostate cancer sufferers should be put on vitamin D3 supplements to reduce the impact of the disease.

Vitamin D3 prevents prostate cancer

In a prospective study from France dated Jan. 28, 2016 a total of 129 prostate cancer cases were diagnosed. The highest quartile versus lowest quartile of 25-hydroxyvitamin D levels were determined. The investigators determined that higher concentrations of 25-hydroxyvitamin D were associated with a decreased risk of prostate cancer. They found that of the group that lived less than 3.3 years on average only 5% survived. On the other hand of the group that survived more than 3.3 years 47% survived.

https://www.ncbi.nlm.nih.gov/pubmed/26568368

Parathyroid hormone is structurally closely related to vitamin D3. However various concentrations of parathyroid hormone showed no effect on prostate cancer occurrence. The authors concluded that in their prospective study vitamin D3 was inversely related to prostate cancer.

Summary: The last two studies show that vitamin D3 cannot only prevent prostate cancer significantly, but it also can lower prostate cancer mortality, once prostate cancer is diagnosed and vit. D3 supplements are taken. As aging men are the ones who develop prostate cancer as a group, they should be taking vitamin D3 supplements in an attempt to reduce the risk to develop prostate cancer or die from it.

10. Lycopene prevents prostate cancer

We all know that lycopenes are high in tomatoes. The Journal of the National Cancer Institute published a report that lycopene prevents prostate cancer.

Lycopenes belong to the carotenoids, which is a group of antioxidant plant chemicals. They are responsible for the red color of tomatoes and other red- pigmented foods.

Regarding this report Harvard researchers looked at data from 49,898 male health professionals. Dietary questionnaires, the number of prostate cancer cases and related deaths have been tracked between 1986 and 2010. The researchers compared the data related to the group with the top 20% of lycopene intake with the data from the group with the bottom 20% of lycopene intake.

There was a 28% lower risk of developing prostate cancer for the group consuming most lycopene when compared to the group consuming the least lycopene. When the risk of lethal prostate cancer was calculated (those who actually died of prostate cancer during the study) the numbers were even more striking: the health care professionals who had the highest intake of lycopenes had a 44% lower risk of dying from prostate cancer than those in the lowest lycopene group. Finally, the researchers looked at early intake of lycopenes versus late start of taking lycopene supplements, and they found that early and ongoing exposure to lycopenes was more protective from prostate cancer. They also found that cancer markers in the blood were lower in the high lycopene group, in particular angiogenesis markers that are responsible for causing prostate cancer to metastasize. The high lycopene group had much less of the substances in the blood that form new blood vessels by a tumor when compared to the low lycopene group; this translated into less prostate cancer metastases and less prostate cancer mortality. So, eat your tomatoes! They are good for prevention of cancer.

Reference: J. Natl. Cancer Inst. 2014 Feb1; 106(2): dj430.

11. Baldness and prostate cancer mortality related

A study from February 2016 by the Johns Hopkins Bloomberg School of Public Health found this fact: baldness and prostate cancer mortality are related.

https://www.ncbi.nlm.nih.gov/pubmed/26764224

Other previous studies have linked prostate cancer and baldness. But this study is the first one to notice that prostate cancer mortality and baldness are related. Prostate cancer mortality is a measure of how many people are killed by prostate cancer. In white men it was a 1.58-fold risk compared to those who were not balding. But previous studies in black men found a slightly higher risk of about a 2.5-fold risk to get prostate cancer when they bald.

Reasons why baldness and prostate cancer mortality are related

Key to baldness and to the development of prostate cancer is the same androgen, dihydrotestosterone (DHT). This is a metabolite of testosterone. It stimulates the prostate to grow in size. It also encourages the transformation of normal prostate cells into prostate cancer cells. DHT also activates male pattern baldness in those men who have inherited the gene that triggers this condition. Many studies have shown that testosterone is NOT the culprit that many have thought it was in the past. To the contrary: it is a LACK of testosterone in aging men what triggers prostate cancer development. Aging men should have their testosterone levels checked and testosterone replaced when those levels are found to be low. On the other hand a male with a history of baldness in the family and coming down himself with baldness has the option of using two medications that have been found to reduce prostate cancer. Proscar (finasteride) and Avodart (dutasteride) have both been shown to reduce the risk of prostate cancer and to reduce the prostate gland volume by 17% to 25% in a relatively short time.

Summary

Don't panic, if you are balding and you hear the threatening message that baldness and prostate cancer mortality are related. But it is important to be vigilant, if you are bald and testosterone deficient at the same time. If you are bald and have testosterone deficiency, you have two risk factors that can cause prostate cancer. You are at a higher risk to get prostate cancer and you should see your physician to make sure your testosterone level is normal. If it is low, ask for testosterone treatment and measure your testosterone level again to make sure it has come up into the high normal range. Next consider Proscar or Avodart and discuss this with your healthcare provider. If you were put on medications like Proscar or Avodart, your DHT level would normalize and your risk to develop prostate cancer would return to normal. Just as a side remark and an example: the philanthropist, Mike Milken is bald and was diagnosed with prostate cancer in 1993.

https://www.bridgespan.org/insights/library/remarkable-givers/profiles/mike-milken/success-story-mike-milken-changes-the-face-of-pr

12. The CaPLESS method

The CaPLESS method is a lifestyle program developed by Dr. Geo Espinoza. He wrote a book about this entitled "Thrive, don't only survive".

http://thrivedontonlysurvive.com/capless-method/

CaPLESS is an acronym: CaP stands for cancer of the prostate, L for lifestyle changes, E for exercise, S for supplementation and the second S for sleep and stress.

Here is the quick 11-point explanation of how to do it:

http://drgeo.com/tag/capless-method-and-prostate-cancer/

1. Become aware of your habits, so you can make lifestyle changes. For instance cut out all sugar and avoid processed foods with sugar in it (read labels). Sugar causes cancer to grow; this is not what you want, so cut sugar out. Exercise regularly and eat fiber regularly.
2. Eat more fruit and vegetables (organic, if possible). You get lots of antioxidant vitamins this way and lignans, all of which fight cancer cells and support your immune system.
3. Do not eat more than 3 to 4 oz. of red meat per week. If you do eat beef, eat grass-fed organic beef. The reason is that there are carcinogens in red meat, more so in regular beef. Eat chicken, turkey and fish instead. In between choose a vegetable dish without any meat. Remember that vegetables also contain protein.

http://www.who.int/features/qa/cancer-red-meat/en/

4. Avoid putting extra salt on your food. There is good evidence that extra salt causes stomach cancer and heart disease:

http://wiki.cancer.org.au/policy/Position_statement_-_Salt_and_cancer_risk

5. Exercise daily for 30 minutes. Work with weights or weight machines twice per week. Exercise reduces prostate cancer.
6. Eat low in calories. A plant-based diet is automatically low in calories.
7. Legumes and grains are good. It is the simple carbs (refined sugar), which are bad for you (cancer causing).
8. Keep your body lean. In other words keep your body mass index low (best between 21 to 22). We talked about the beer-belly before. You can also buy body composition scales and measure your fat percentage that way.

http://www.builtlean.com/2010/08/03/ideal-body-fat-percentage-chart/

9. Supplements were mentioned above. We had talked about vitamin D3, take at least 5000 IU per day. Fiber intake halves your prostate cancer risk. Also, think about eating more tomatoes because they contain cancer- fighting lycopenes.
10. There is one more point I like to raise: Have your testosterone level checked; if it is below 500 ng/dl (= 17.3 nmol/l), see your doctor for a bioidentical testosterone cream or for testosterone shots. Contrary to all of the dire warnings of conventional medicine about testosterone being dangerous, the opposite of what they say is true. Young men don't get prostate cancer, because they have very high testosterone levels. Older men with testosterone replacement also don't get prostate cancer, but older men with deficient testosterone levels do. Dr. Geo Espinoza did not mention bioidentical hormone replacement, but I did. Testosterone prevents strokes, heart attacks and prostate cancer. Every year

when I go to the Annual World Congress on Anti-Aging Medicine (mid December) in Las Vegas the fact that low testosterone causes prostate cancer is mentioned by several speakers. And they also mention that when testosterone is low, it needs to be replaced.

11. Manage your sleep and watch your stress management! When you get enough sleep, and you handle stress well, your immune system functions better. Your hormones are more balanced, and you have more energy. This allows you to fight cancer better, wounds heal better and your cardiovascular state is in good shape. If you have too many commitments, you may need to cut some of them out to help manage your stress. You may have to learn to say "no" to avoid overcommitments.

13. Prognosis after prostate cancer surgery

Physicians have researched for a long time what kind of life expectancy a man would have after a certain prostate cancer stage was diagnosed. The earlier prostate cancer is detected, the better the long-term outlook. If there are metastases at the time of the diagnosis, the prognosis is poor. In chapter 4 I have displayed a table regarding the average 5-year and 10-year survivals with prostate cancer. As already indicated how long you will live depends very much on what lifestyle you have. As I have discussed above, if you follow a balanced diet, exercise and take some supplements, you will live longer. If you grow a beer belly, you have an estrogen factory in your fatty tissue due to the enzyme aromatase. Aromatase takes testosterone and turns it into estrogen, which shortens your life span. Too much estrogen can make prostate cancer come back. Too much estrogen can even cause more prostate cancer by converting harmless prostate cells into prostate cancer cells.

As a result the long-term survival after prostate cancer has been diagnosed is very much dependent on the lifestyle of the patient. If you have a high or rising PSA and you see your doctor right away about this, a mapping biopsy will establish whether prostate cancer is present. It will also tell you whether there is only one focus or several foci and whether it is localized. If this is treated with ablation cryotherapy, you will have a high probability that this is the end of the prostate cancer. Your prognosis should be close to 100% that you will be around in 10 years from now. In the meantime by optimizing your lifestyle as described above, you will improve your life expectancy even further. You can now say: Prostate cancer is unmasked and you can control this once mysterious disease.

Conclusion

There are many factors that help to prevent prostate cancer. The effect of prevention is something that is easier to measure in a population; prevention is still effective in an individual case, but is more difficult to prove. Nevertheless the factors discussed above will help you to have a lower probability of a cancer recurrence after your prostate cancer treatment is done. It is never too late for positive lifestyle changes! What are the major beneficial factors?

- If you are smoking, quit smoking. The carcinogens in the cigarette smoke would stimulate the prostate cancer stem cells to multiply. This is not what you want.
- If you have a beer belly, lose weight because the estrogen that is produced through the enzyme aromatase will cause more cancer. It will do this also after your surgery or radiation therapy. I have discussed this above where I mentioned the M.D. Anderson Cancer Center in Houston, Texas study.

- Have a balanced diet like a Mediterranean diet. Avoid sugar; it stimulates cancer growth.
- Don't exceed moderate alcohol consumption.
- Take extra vitamin D3 in the order of 5000 IU per day. It stimulates your immune system and makes the cancer weaker.
- Exercise regularly. This makes you stronger and stimulates your immune system.
- If your testosterone is below 500 ng/dl (= 17.3 nmol/l), see your doctor for a bioidentical testosterone cream or for testosterone shots. Testosterone is your friend, not your enemy. I have discussed this in detail in chapter 7. Your body cells have testosterone receptors that need stimulation from testosterone; this will keep your body healthy.

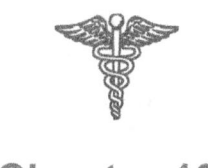

Chapter 19

Differential Diagnosis: Prostatitis & Benign Prostatic Hyperplasia (BPH)

When the clinician listens to the symptoms of a patient and examines him, the doctor thinks about alternative diagnoses, called "differential diagnoses". Could the symptoms and findings fit a diagnosis of prostatitis, an enlargement of the prostate (BPH) or prostate cancer? Here I like to briefly review the two conditions that are different from prostate cancer: prostatitis and benign prostatic hyperplasia (also called benign prostatic hypertrophy or BPH).

Prostatitis

This condition is an inflammation of the prostate gland. Only about 5 to 10% of cases are thought to be due to a bacterial infection. In older males an enlarged prostate gland (BPH) is often associated with prostatitis. If a male has problems with urinary flow and uses self-catheterization this too can cause prostatitis.

Otherwise a recent bladder infection or an abnormality in the urinary tract can cause prostatitis as well. Prostatitis is not causing prostate cancer.

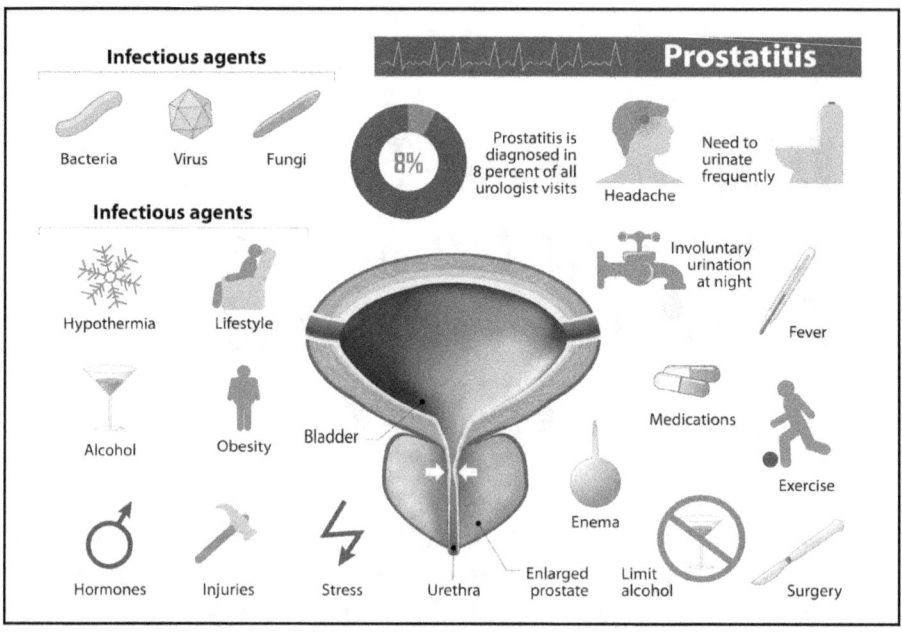

Symptoms of prostatitis

A man with acute prostatitis often has frequent urination and urgency. Urination may be painful, and it can be difficult to pass urine. Increased urination at night can cause disrupted sleep. There is pelvic pain and pain in the genital area.

There may even be rectal pain with defecation, as the rectum is situated right behind the prostate gland. If the cause is bacterial, there may be a high fever and chills, nausea and vomiting. Other symptoms can be pains that come and go in the lower mid abdomen. There may be pain around the anus, in the groin on both sides or in the lower back. There could be pain with sexual intercourse as the prostate contracts a bit during ejaculation. These are all symptoms that should send the patient to a doctor! Otherwise his partner may drag him to the doctor's office.

Treatment

An acute prostatitis can escalate into an emergency! When the patient has pains, chills and a fever he needs treatment in the hospital setting with intravenous fluids, antibiotics and pain medications.

Chronic prostatitis

A man with frequent urine infections may initially be unaware that his prostate is being infected. Symptoms are not as pronounced as with acute prostatitis, and this can be the reason that often the diagnosis is delayed. Treatment for chronic bacterial prostatitis consists of long-term antibiotics, given for 4 to 12 weeks.

Some cases require ongoing low-dose antibiotic treatment to help control symptoms.

Chronic nonbacterial prostatitis

When no bacterial cause can be found by repeat urinary cultures, but prostatitis symptoms are present, chronic nonbacterial prostatitis is diagnosed. Alternatively this is also called chronic pelvic pain syndrome. About 90% of chronic prostatitis cases belong into this category. A patient with this condition usually had pelvic and genital pain for at least 3 months of the past 6 months.

Even though some urologists state that bacterial infections are rare, others say that Trichomonas vaginalis, Chlamydia trachomatis, genital mycoplasmas, staphylococci, coryneforms, and genital viruses can also cause prostatitis. However, these are much more difficult to culture or document.

Diagnostic tests

One way to overcome the poor documentation of prostatitis with a simple urine culture is to do a double urine culture. The physician or specialist collects a midstream urine sample first, then does a prostate massage through a rectal examination and repeats another midstream urine sample for culture and sensitivity testing. With prostatitis there will often be negative or light growth with the pre prostate massage urine sample and a denser growth of bacteria in the post prostate massage urine sample. In this case there is proof of a chronic prostatitis. The bacteria can be deeply buried in prostatic tissue, and only a prostate massage will release some for culture.

In chronic cases a referral to an urologist is required. The specialist may decide that a prostate biopsy needs to be done to look at the tissue histologically.

In a study, 135 men were described with chronic prostatitis that did not respond to multiple antibiotic courses. In 8% of them there were positive tests of Mycoplasma genitalium, Chlamydia trachomatis, or Trichomonas vaginalis by PCR assay (Polymerase chain reaction).

https://en.wikipedia.org/wiki/Polymerase_chain_reaction)

This genetic test is much more sensitive than conventional culture procedures and picks up traces of

DNA from bacteria. In 25% of this group of 135 men with chronic prostatitis broad-spectrum PCR tests were positive for other bacteria.

This data suggests that the prostate can harbor bacteria in its tissue that are not easily detectable using conventional urine cultures.

What these studies have shown is that it is the safest to go by the patient's symptoms. If chronic symptoms are there, very likely one or more of these infectious agents are present. This means that this patient needs to be referred to an urologist for a possible transperineal prostate biopsy and a more prolonged treatment.

Enlarged prostate gland: Benign Prostatic Hyperplasia (BPH)

We don't know why, but aging men often have an enlargement of their prostate gland. This can cause problems urinating because the prostate capsule around the prostate gland is relatively stiff. As the prostate gland expands inside the prostatic capsule, pressure is exerted onto the urethra that crosses through the prostate gland. This creates problems with the urinary stream. It takes a lot longer for the man to empty his bladder. About 50% of men above the age of 75 are affected to a greater or lesser degree by symptoms of BPH.

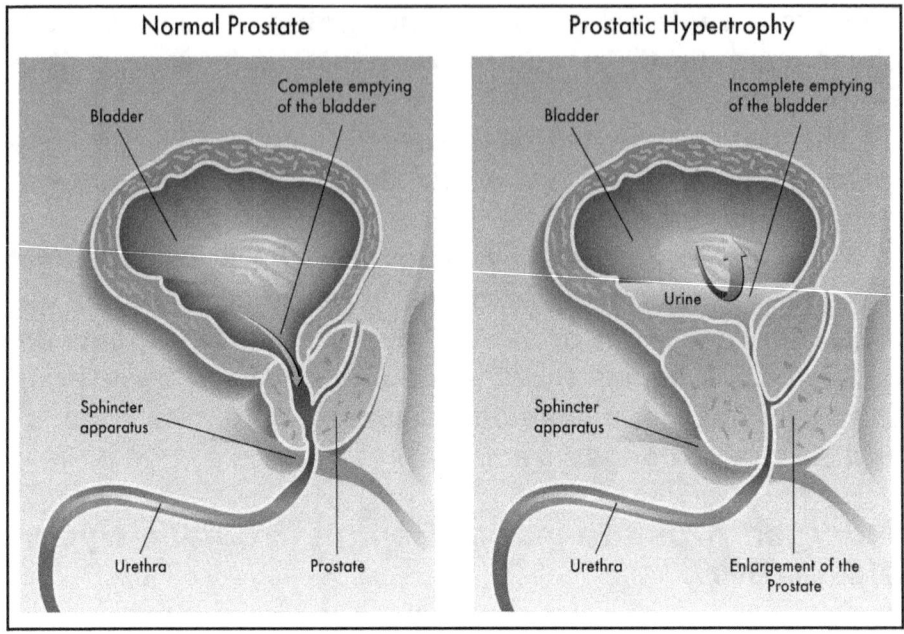

| Normal Prostate | Prostatic Hypertrophy |

Symptoms of BPH

There can be difficulties starting the urinary stream, having decreased strength of the urinary stream or dribbling at the end of urination. The patient with BPH may feel that the bladder is not completely emptied. It may be painful to urinate and there may be an urge to urinate again shortly after urination was completed. Other symptoms are waking frequently at night to urinate or having an uncontrollable urge to urinate. During the day a patient with BPH will urinate more often than was the case in the past.

Diagnostic tests

In order to find out whether a man with BPH retains urine in the bladder, a simple ultrasound investigation can assess the bladder before emptying and repeat the ultrasound examination following the emptying of the bladder again. The ultrasound can measure the residual urine in the bladder. A post void residual volume (PVR) of less than 50 ml is acceptable in a person younger than 65.

Above the age of 65 a PVR of less than 100 ml is acceptable.

A rectal examination is not reliable in terms of estimating the size of the prostate. An MRI scan is much more reliable to measure the total volume of the prostate gland and whether or not prostate hypertrophy is present. A volume of less than 25 cubic centimeters is normal. This paper explains that based on the MRI findings one can define 7 different BPH types depending on where the enlargement is centered.

https://www.ncbi.nlm.nih.gov/pmc/articles/PMC4859736/

Another advantage is that an MRI scan can help to confirm that prostate cancer is absent. Although BPH does not cause prostate cancer, it sometimes can be difficult to diagnose an early prostate cancer in a large prostate gland. Also, the PSA test that is used to screen for prostate cancer can be elevated when the prostate gland is enlarged, which makes it difficult on its own merit to rule out prostate cancer as the cause of the elevated PSA.

Treatment of BPH

1. Mild cases of BPH: Double voiding can treat milder cases of BPH. The patient is encouraged to urinate as much as possible. After waiting for a few moments he should void again. Avoid caffeine and alcohol as they increase the urge to urinate. Avoid medicines that interfere with bladder emptying, such as antihistamines and decongestants. Saw palmetto or beta-sitosterol are herbal medicines that can help with mild cases of BPH.

2. **More severe cases of BPH:** For more serious cases it goes without saying that an urologist should be consulted. In all likelihood a medication will be prescribed. There is the group of alpha-blockers like terazosin (Hytrin). This tends to improve urination and urinary retention within 3 months. But unfortunately one of the side effects is erectile dysfunction. Others are drowsiness, a stuffy or runny nose, blurred or hazy vision; nausea, swelling or puffiness in hands, feet, or lower legs.

a) There are other drugs that can be useful, for instance the 5-alpha reductase inhibitors. Two common drugs that belong into this group are: finasteride (Proscar) and dutasteride (Avodart). The side effect of these are erectile dysfunction, but both Proscar and Avodart work very well in reducing the prostate gland size and in improving BPH symptoms. Avodart, the newer of the two, works faster.

b) The FDA has accepted the phosphodiesterase-5 (PDE-5) inhibitor tadalafil (Cialis) as a treatment for BPH. Of course the original indication for Cialis is erectile dysfunction. But the fact that the sexual performance improves with this drug and it helps at the same time to reduce the prostate size, is a very useful combination of effects. Many patients with BPA have erectile dysfunction, so they benefit from Cialis in these two ways. Should the physician choose to put a patient on Hytrin or on Avodart, this could also be combined with Cialis. This way the side effect of erectile dysfunction of these other drugs would be treated at the same time as bladder and urination functions improve.

c) If all these methods do not help, the urologist may suggest a minor surgical procedure. The less surgery is performed, the better the result will be, as there is less scarring. With the transurethral incision of the prostate (TUIP) some tissue is removed from within the prostate gland in the area of the bladder neck. Cutting one or two small grooves into the urinary channel to allow urine to flow more freely will achieve this. This newer method is a lot better tolerated than the older method of transurethral resection of the prostate (TURP). Another surgical procedure is the transurethral microwave therapy (TUMT), where microwave energy is used to destroy part of the prostate gland, which reduces the pressure on the urethra. With the transurethral needle ablation surgery (TUNA) a heated needle is used to remove some of the prostatic tissue. None of these procedures have been around long enough to be able to say what the long-term outcomes will be. In a 2012 publication the use of laser is also mentioned for treating BPH and bladder obstruction.

https://uroweb.org/wp-content/uploads/Herrmann-Th.-et-al-Eur-Urol-2012-614783-EAU-Guidelines-on-laser-technologies.pdf

d) Another paper describes the use of laser to vaporize tissue in the case of BPH.

https://www.ncbi.nlm.nih.gov/pubmed/20035978

Considering the effects of the newer drugs like dutasteride (Avodart) and tadalafil (Cialis) there is now less of a need for surgical procedures. Also, the surgical procedures have been minimized, which helps in terms of reducing the untoward side effects of the surgical procedures.

Conclusion about prostatitis and BPH

Men can have non-cancerous prostate conditions. The most common ones are prostatitis and BPH. With prostatitis there is an acute or chronic inflammation in the prostate. As the infection can hide in the prostate gland, it may be difficult to get a bacterial culture through a urine culture test. Sometimes low dose prolonged antibiotic therapy is required for this condition.

Benign prostatic hyperplasia (BPH) is a common condition in aging males. It often becomes manifest only when the man has a problem voiding. The urethra can get obstructed as it crosses through an enlarged prostate gland. There are several remedies that have been found that help reduce the size of the prostate gland. These have been described in detail above. Cialis helps both erectile dysfunction and BPH and can be useful for these men, as they often have problems with erectile dysfunction as well.

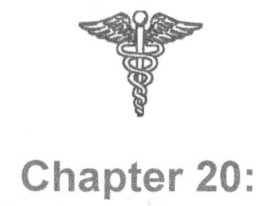

Chapter 20:

Prostate Cancer Support Groups

Here is a link to information about prostate cancer support groups:

https://www.pcf.org/c/finding-a-support-group/

If you are insecure about what to do, you may get answers from some of these groups. But be careful that you are not talked into something that you do not want to be part of.

I joined one of these support groups that I found on the Internet and it seemed that everybody was very hot on "active surveillance". When I stated that I felt the cancer should be removed with ablation cryotherapy right away, I was criticized. Everybody was very opinionated; one said only laser ablation therapy would be the method to use. Another said that the gold standard of therapy would be radical prostatectomy. They did not want to know about the mapping biopsy. This is when I quit the group. I have never heard from them again.

Nobody but you yourself owns your prostate cancer problem. In this book I pointed out what methods exist to remove the cancer safely. I explained what I did and why. But you need to decide for yourself what will work for you. No support group can do that for you. It is important to read everything to be able to make an informed decision. But if you allow a support group to lull you into the belief that it would be safe to go on active surveillance instead of intervening with the prostate cancer right away, this undue influence could cost you your life within 10 years or earlier.

How to approach advanced prostate cancer

When the patient reaches stage IV of prostate cancer there can be metastases in the pelvic area. This could include the lymph glands, but may also involve metastases in the pelvic bone. The cancer may also have spread into the lower back (lymph glands and bone). Metastases may have found their way into the lungs, liver and into the brain.

It is very unlikely that either radiation, chemotherapy or hormone ablation therapy will slow down the growth of the cancer at this stage.

Conventional medicine has nothing to offer to this end-stage prostate cancer patient except supportive care with pain medication.

Dr. Onik whose work I described in chapter 15, has a different idea. He is now concentrating on end-stage prostate cancer patients.

In this case he would still be doing a mapping biopsy, because he can see where the tumor is located in the prostate gland. This area is treated with ablation cryotherapy, because the therapy kills a sizeable amount of the original cancer and stimulates the immune system to produce antibodies directed at the cancer and prostate cancer stem cells. Killer T-cells also attack the tumor. At the present time he has achieved a cure rate of 30% in these hopeless end-stage prostate cancer patients, for whom there would otherwise not be any hope. With other patients there may be a partial improvement, but in the remainder of patients there will not be any change. However, with conventional medicine 100% of these end stage patients die. With Dr. Onik's method at least 30% are cured and some live a few months or years longer.

At this stage there is nothing better available. Hopefully the future will improve the immune therapy approach.

Here is a link how to approach the end stage of prostate cancer when nothing helps:

https://www.cancer.org/content/cancer/en/search.html?q= treatment+nearing+the+end+of+life

There are hospice facilities where end stage cancer patients can turn to, if they can't cope at home. Counseling is also often helpful to come to terms with issues of death and dying.

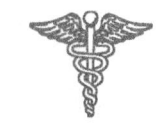

Chapter 21

Conclusion: What Does It Mean to Unmask Prostate Cancer?

The key with prostate cancer, like with any cancer, is early diagnosis. If you catch prostate cancer at stage 1 or early stage 2 there is a good chance that prostate surgery will be able to eradicate the entire tumor. But it is important to choose the right surgical method. Although a form of radical prostatectomy (conventional, laparoscopic or robotic) is considered to be the gold standard of prostate surgery, I do not think that this is the wisest choice. It only has a 10-year survival rate of 77% in the Johns Hopkins study that I mentioned.

A laser ablation surgery is also not optimal as it can damage the neurovascular bundle and can lead to urinary incontinence, if the bladder outlet is injured. Also, this is a relatively new procedure and 10-year survival trials have not yet been done. The patient becomes part of an ongoing trial, but I'm no so sure that you want to be a human test case with no guarantees attached!

In my opinion Dr. Onik's method of ablation cryotherapy in combination with the NanoKnife (=IRE surgery) is the best combination. It is done under rectal ultrasonography control and is based on the pathological findings from the mapping biopsy. This procedure removes all of the histologically proven cancer tissues, but preserves the neurovascular bundles, which are important for pre-servation of the urinary and sexual functions. It also preserves the seminal vesicles and the healthy prostatic glandular tissue, which preserves healthy ejaculations. This is important for sexual rehabilitation.

In addition the cancer vaccination aspect of both cryotherapy and IRE surgery that eradicate the prostate cancer stem cells (CSC) is important to prevent recurrences of the cancer. None of the standard methods like radical prostatectomy, hormone deprivation therapy, radiotherapy and chemotherapy are addressing this aspect of the prostate cancer therapy. As explained above the surface antigens of the killed cancer cells are the same as the ones of the CSC's and antibody formation and killer cell formation from the ablation cryotherapy and IRE surgery will automatically eradicate the cancer stem cells.

The intriguing feature of unmasking prostate cancer is the possibility of doing cancer surgery through the perineum without any visible scar. The rectal approach is avoided, as it has the risk of E.coli infection. There is minimal interference with the patient's life style as the procedures (mapping biopsy and ablation cryotherapy/IRE surgery) are done on a daycare surgery basis. The surgery has the built-in cancer vaccination aspect as explained. This ensures to a large extent that there will be no cancer recurrence. Three to five months later the patient's sex life will return to normal, once the irritation from the prostate procedure wears off. It really is the best treatment option with the highest survival rate of 100% at the 10-year follow-up point. Of the patients treated 94% were completely free from any recurring prostate cancer. This is based on low PSA values at the 10-year point following the ablation cryotherapy procedure. Only 6% had recurring disease, but these patients were alive. These were the best survival figures, when I researched the various treatment modalities.

It occurred to me that there are several hidden truths that are easily overlooked. I had to dig into 10-year survival figures to unearth which method of treating prostate cancer would be best.

We discussed these figures already, but here they are summarized again to refresh your memory:

- Laparoscopic prostatectomy has a 10-year survival rate of only 77% (Johns Hopkins study). All other variations of radical prostatectomy have similar 10-year survivals. A Swiss study was cited with a 10-year survival rate of 98%. Another study from New York showed a 10-year survival of 99% for the medium risk group and 88.5% for the high-risk group.
- Brachytherapy at 10 years: the Georgia Center reported that 57 % had a PSA of less than 0.2, which means that the cure rate is only 57%!
- Hormone ablation therapy alone: 11-year survival 77%.
- Hormone ablation and radiotherapy after 11 years: 90%.
- Proton radiation therapy: 10-year survival rates (Loma Linda University Medical Center) were 73%.
- High-intensity focused ultrasound (HIFU): survival at 10 years was 61%.
- Ablation cryotherapy: highest survival rate of 100% at the 10-year follow-up point. 94% of the patients treated with ablation cryotherapy were completely free from any recurring prostate cancer, but in 6% the PSA was elevated.

As we compare survival rates and complication rates at 10 years between the various options of prostate cancer treatment, it is clear that there are differences that can be unmasked. In my opinion this is the way to compare the success rates of the various procedures.

Conventional cancer medicine does not take into consideration that there are cancer stem cells in any cancer and in particular in prostate cancer. If this is ignored, there will be recurrences of tumors because prostate cancer stem cells are radioresistant and chemotherapy resistant. It would be useful to avoid radiotherapy, because this way we avoid creating radioresistant cancer cells, which likely is the cause of the high recurrence rates of prostate cancer within 5 years of brachytherapy treatment. Surgery and cryoablation therapy are methods that remove prostate cancer stem cells. This is another fact that was unmasked in this book.

Dr. Gary Onik is utilizing the knowledge of prostate cancer stem cells to vaccinate against the patient's own tumor as he performs the cryoablation therapy. His procedure achieves both: it eliminates the cancer cells and vaccinates against the cancer to allow the immune system to remove the last cancer cells.

The patients who become positive for PSA following cryoablation therapy have an option of repeating the same procedure again. A repeat mapping biopsy and cryoablation therapy has a high probability of eradicating the recurrent prostate cancer. This is not something that is offered by any other treatment technique. And doing ablation following radical prostatectomy or following radiotherapy would be very difficult to do because of the extensive scarring in the treatment area. Here is another mask that has been removed.

"**Prostate cancer unmasked**" **simply means to use all of the information that I provided in this book and making an informed decision, which treatment is best to follow. I hope it will work for you as it did for me.**

Index

V

Vitamin D3 XXVii, 56, 150, 151, 163, 164, 169, 172

Vitamins Xii, XXVii, 56, 149-151, 163, 164, 168, 169, 172

W

Watchful waiting XiX, 5, 58, 61, 62

Westernized diet 158, 159

X

X chromosome, 27, 160

Xenoestrogens 47, 158

Y

Yellow laser light (589 nm) 103

Z

Zyflamend 56